AF886172

# EYEFACETS

Written by T. David Williams



Published by Creative Connex Inc.

Cover by Alise Fife

ISBN: 978-1-0693418-0-8

Printed in Canada

First Edition



COVER PHOTO : View of living cornea, photographed with slit lamp (author's collection).

# FOREWORD

The author of this book, T. David Williams, and I, have known each other since 1968 when I arrived at Indiana University to pursue a graduate degree (he was a couple of years ahead of me).

We ended up in lengthy academic careers at the same place, the University of Waterloo, School of Optometry and Vision Science. This book is a distillation of David's many years in research and teaching.

The book is only 242 pages long, and that includes a 27-page glossary. Amazingly, it also includes 177 figures, both photographs and drawings, all with simply and clearly worded captions. The many original drawings supplement the text. They clarify the anatomical characteristics of the structures of the eye and the neuronal pathways that carry visual information to the brain.

In spite of its size, this book includes everything: Anatomy and physiology of the eye and the visual pathways, colour vision, the eye's optical characteristics, and a summary of possible refractive errors and their correction. It also includes descriptions of what can go wrong. The topics covered include, for example, dry eye, macular degeneration, glaucoma and cataract, and the effects of systemic problems, such as diabetes and hypertension.

As a compact description of the eye and the issues that affect ocular health this book is a tour de force. A possible sub-title might be 'Everything you wanted to know about the eye and were afraid to ask".

**Jacob Sivak**
Distinguished Professor Emeritus, University of Waterloo

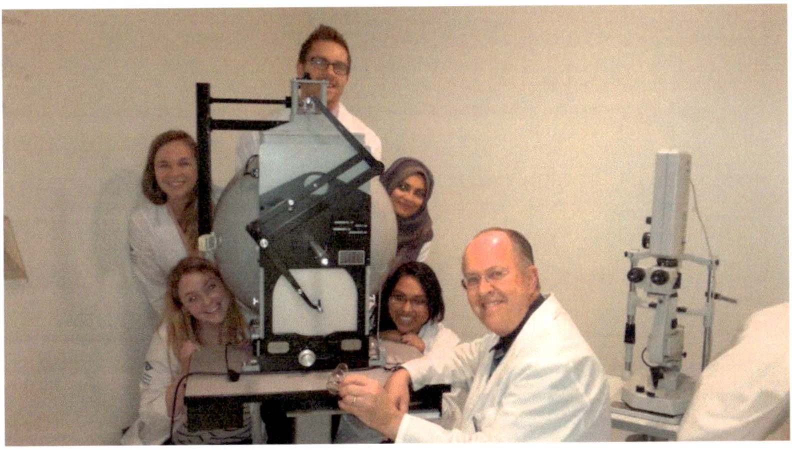

ABOUT THE AUTHOR

Dr. T. David Williams holds a Doctor of Optometry degree (College of Optometry of Ontario), Master of Science (Indiana University), and Ph.D. (Indiana University). He is a Professor Emeritus of the School of Optometry and Vision Science, University of Waterloo, Ontario, Canada, where he taught in the areas of general and ocular disease (among others) and authored 158 publications. This book is based on 50 years of clinical experience related to the eye and eye problems.

PREFACE

I have written this book to provide basic information about the eye and vision. As you look through it, I hope you find a number of facts that surprise you and illuminate the wonders of this magnificent organ. You will also be impressed by how small the parts of the eye are, and why the eye is really a part of the brain which has wandered out of the skull. A tour through the eye will take you through its embryonic development, how it works, and why we sometimes see things that aren't there, and other times fail to see others which *are* there.

# Contents

# Chapter 1 PARTS OF THE EYE

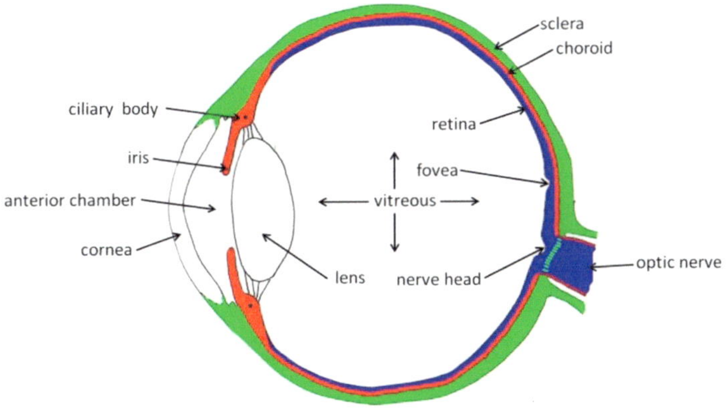


Figure 1 Parts of the eye

Before getting into a discussion of the parts of the eye, it is helpful to spend a moment considering methods of examination of these parts. The premier instrument for examining the eye is the slit lamp, which combines a fine binocular microscope with an ingenious light source. This combination permits examination of all parts of the eye. The cornea and lens may be seen in optical sections: a thin sheet of light directed at an angle into the eye allows the examiner to see a slice of the living cornea or lens in great detail. (Details on the slit lamp are in Figure 155 in the section on Cataract.) The use of additional lenses allows a view of the eye at any point between the front of the eye and the back of the eye. A special contact lens (the gonioscope shown in Figure 3) permits examination of the angle of the anterior chamber, and also of the extreme periphery of the retina.

A second type of instrument is useful for studying the retina and optic nerve head: this may be either the direct or indirect ophthalmoscope. Each has its unique advantages: the direct ophthalmoscope allows a high-magnification (15x) view of retinal and nerve head details over a relatively small area (around 5 degrees wide), while the indirect ophthalmoscope allows a low-magnification (5x) view over a wider area (about 30 degrees wide). The optics of both ophthalmoscopes will be discussed later in the section on REFRACTION, Figures 82 and 83.

## CORNEA

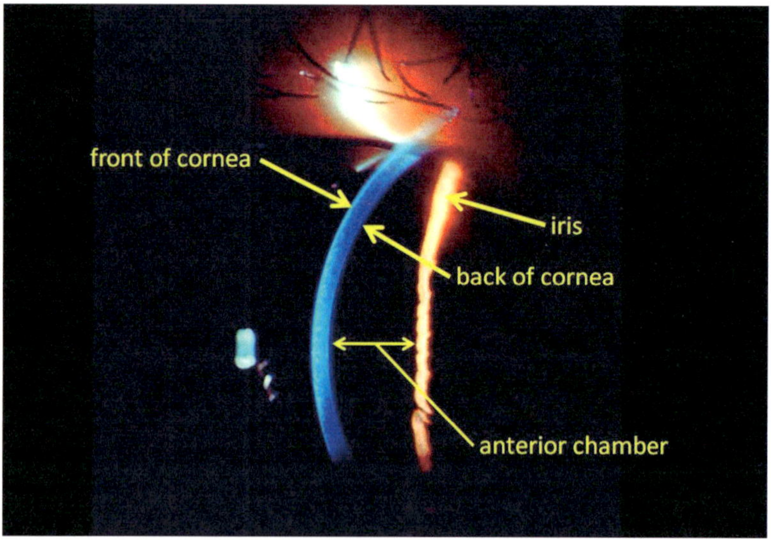


**Figure 2 Optical section of cornea, showing anterior chamber**

Here is a slit lamp view of the cornea. You can see the thickness of the cornea in this optical slice. Although the cornea is only half a millimeter thick at its center, the microscope can focus accurately on all layers. The cornea becomes thicker as it approaches the join between cornea and sclera (the limbus). Because the thin vertical beam of light also hits the iris, you can get a sense of the depth of the anterior chamber, which is usually around 3 millimeters.

The cornea is continuous with the opaque white of the eye (SCLERA); however, the corneal structure is more regular than the sclera and has less water in it because of the pumping action of the endothelium which lines the cornea on the anterior chamber side. These factors are necessary for the cornea to be transparent. The sclera, on the other hand, has lots of water in it, and is opaque. With its high curvature, the cornea provides 45 diopters of the total focal power (60 diopters) of the eye. The rest of the focal power comes from the lens, which contributes some 15 diopters. This high-powered optical system is needed in order to focus images at the retina, which is a mere 16 mm from the back of the lens.

The outermost part of the cornea is the epithelium, while the stroma makes up the bulk of the corneal thickness. Within the stroma are keratocytes, which can transform into fibroblasts and/or phagocytic cells should they be needed. The tough, elastic membrane of Descemet lies at the bottom of the stroma, and the single layer of endothelial cells lies on the anterior chamber side of Descemet membrane. The cornea is bathed by tears on one side, and aqueous humor on the other. The tears and the aqueous humor have compositions similar to the blood, so if there are high levels of lipids or other materials, they may be deposited in the cornea.

The hexagonal cells of the corneal endothelium are 0.5 micrometers thick and 20 micrometers wide. At the boundary between sclera and cornea (the limbus), dozens of nerve fibers enter the corneal epithelium. These nerves are very fine and only visible with magnification at the slit lamp where they look as fine as spider web. Fine loops of blood vessels ring the cornea at the limbus: these may enlarge in cases of corneal infection. Larger blood vessels may invade the cornea should stronger defences against infection be needed.

## ANTERIOR CHAMBER

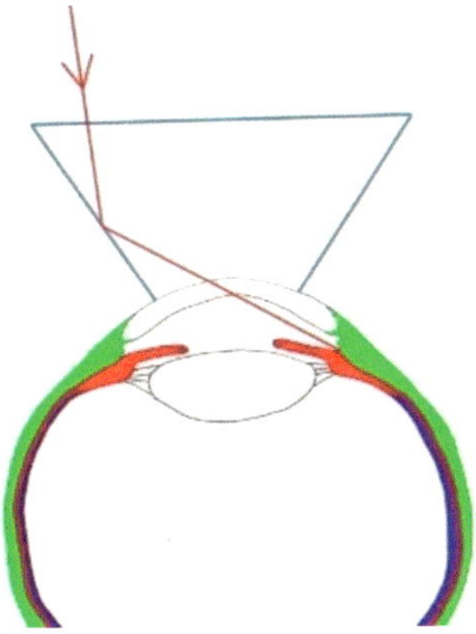

**Figure 3 gonioscope**

A special contact lens with a mirror (a gonioscope, shown in Fig. 3) is required to permit the view shown in Figure 4. This contact lens is placed on the cornea with a layer of gel between it and the cornea. Because the plastic of the gonioscope, the gel, and the cornea itself all have nearly the same refractive index, the light from the slit lamp bounces off the mirrored side of the gonioscope directly into the anterior chamber without being bent at all.

The ANTERIOR CHAMBER is bounded by the lens and iris posteriorly, and the cornea anteriorly. The Anterior chamber angle runs around its periphery. The chamber is filled with aqueous humor, which is secreted by the ciliary body, permeates the vitreous, and passes out of the eye at the anterior chamber angle. Some of the aqueous humor also passes across the sclera.

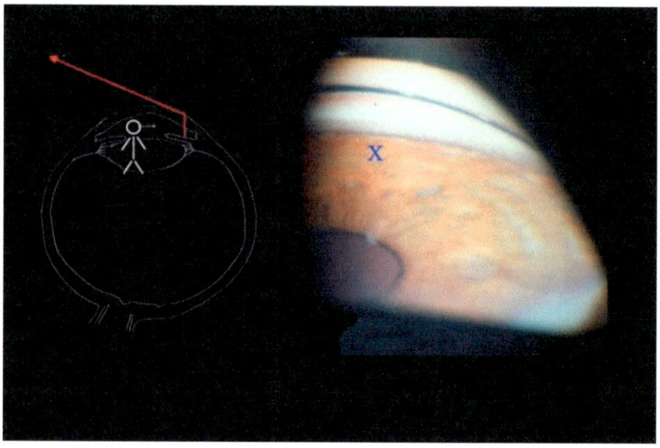


**Figure 4 Anterior chamber angle details**

There is a steady turnover of aqueous humor, similar to the turnover of cerebrospinal fluid within the brain. The depth of the anterior chamber in a young person is around 3 millimeters, but decreases with age as the lens thickens. In cases of inflammation within the eye, cells may invade the anterior chamber, where they may be seen floating in the beam of the slit lamp. These cells may be removed by the body's phagocytic cells, or they may become deposited on the back surface of the cornea, or in the anterior chamber angle, where they may impede the outflow of aqueous.

On the right of Fig. 4 is a view of the Anterior chamber angle of the eye, the space lying between the root of the iris and the outer structures of the eye.

The stick figure on the left of Fig. 4 shows the viewpoint for the clinical image on the right of Figure 4. Starting at the edge of the pupil, you can see along the surface of the iris, and note a darker brown band at the far end of the iris, where it is attached to the ciliary body. Above that brown band, you can see a grayish band, and then, higher still, a band of white. The grayish band is where fluid drains out of the eye. The white band is sclera. Light travelling from the point marked 'X' will just escape the eye, as it strikes the cornea at the critical angle (shown with red arrow). Light from any structures further into the angle than the point 'X' will be reflected at the cornea so these structures cannot be seen when you look normally at the eye. The most peripheral 2.2 millimeters of the anterior chamber are not visible. In other words, the iris is 4.4 millimeters wider than it appears and does not end at the visible join between the cornea and the sclera (the limbus).

## IRIS

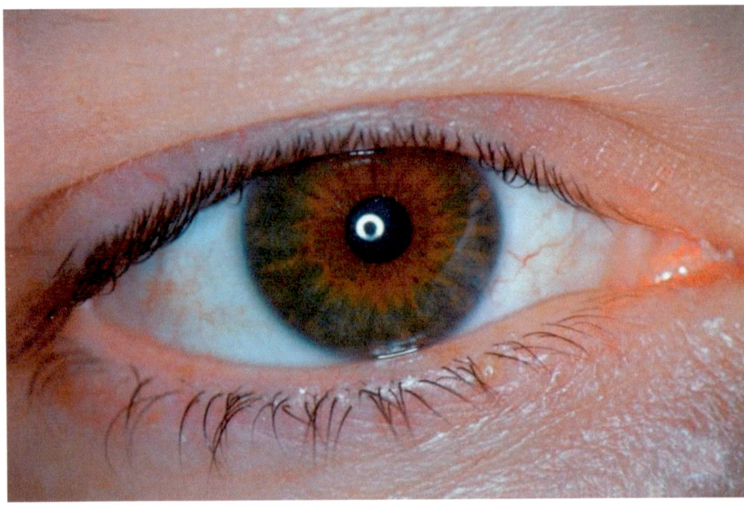

Figure 5 Hazel iris

The iris is the coloured part of the eye. Like the ciliary body, the iris is highly vascular. It has two sets of muscles: one to cause the pupil to dilate, the other to cause the pupil to constrict. When you look at a nearby object, the pupil constricts, the ciliary muscle contracts, and the lens assumes a more curved shape: this is accommodation. Prolonged contraction of the ciliary muscle may cause discomfort. The iris has four layers: the two front layers contain varying amounts of pigment (which determines eye colour), while the two back layers are heavily pigmented and are formed from the two layers at the rim of the embryonic optic cup.

## CILIARY BODY

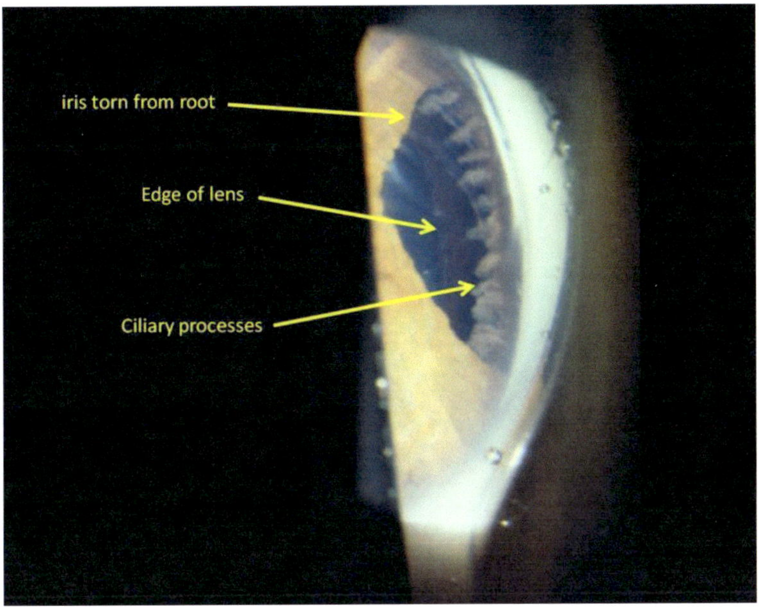


**Figure 6 Gonioscope view of ciliary processes**

The ciliary body is highly vascular and secretes aqueous humor via the ciliary processes, which lie behind the iris. The ciliary processes are not normally visible, but because of an injury to this eye, the root of the iris separated from the ciliary body. Using the gonioscope, we can see through this window.

The ciliary processes are tufts of blood vessels attached to the ciliary body and extending toward the vitreous. The lens is also anchored to the ciliary body. The vitreous has its strongest attachment at the ciliary body. When the circular ciliary muscle contracts, the tension on the lens is reduced and it tends to assume a rounder shape, particularly on its front surface.

# LENS

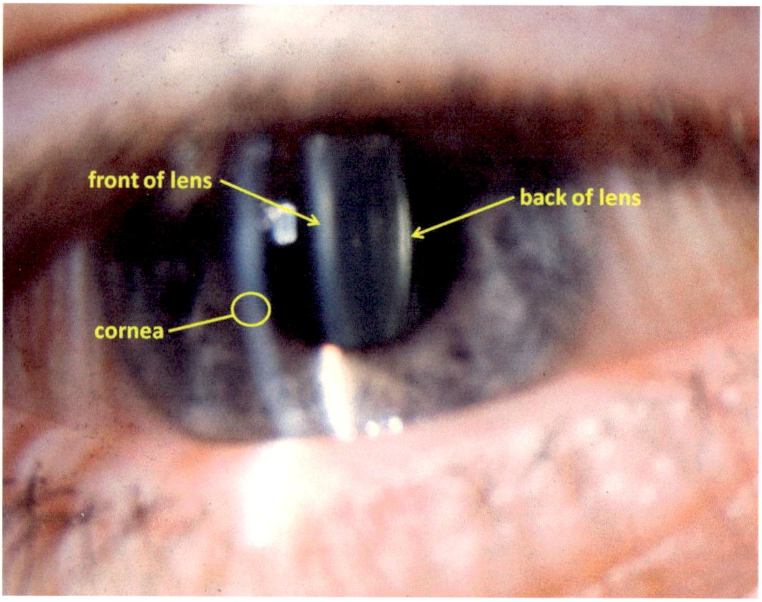


Figure 7 Optical sections of lens

Here is a slit lamp view of the lens, with the focus on the posterior surface of the lens. The lens is derived from ectoderm, as are the skin and corneal epithelium. From the early days of anatomy, the lens has been called the CRYSTALLINE LENS. Early anatomists were so impressed by its jewel-like quality that for some time the crystalline lens was thought to be the place where vision happened. While layers of skin rise to the surface and fall off, the layers of the lens move inwards toward the core of the lens.

The lens in a 10 year old is 3 millimeters thick, and 6 millimeters thick in an 80 year old. A young lens is flexible, so it can take on steeper curves to increase its focal power and allow the seeing of nearby objects. With age, the thicker lens becomes less flexible. This explains some of the problems older people have with seeing up close. The focal power of the lens is roughly 15 diopters. Because of the pigment in the retina and choroid, the eye acts as a light trap, which is why you cannot ordinarily see the lens. Many fine fibers from the ciliary body are attached to the lens capsule around its perimeter, suspending it just behind the iris. This system of fibers is referred to as the zonule.

## VITREOUS

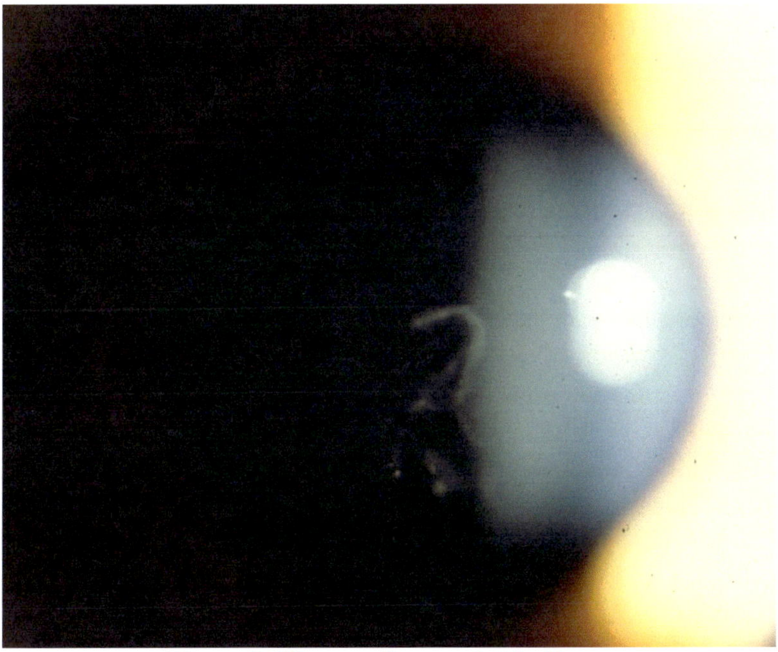

**Figure 8 Vitreous floaters behind lens**

The distance from the lens to the retina is 16 millimeters. The rear 2/3 of the eyeball is filled with a jelly-like, clear material called VITREOUS HUMOR or, more simply, VITREOUS. This slit lamp view is focused just behind the posterior surface of the lens. The vitreous is mostly water, hyaluronic acid, and some strands of collagen. Over time, these collagen strands may clump together and become large enough to be seen against an open sky or white wall (vitreous floaters).

At four months after conception, the vitreous space is largely occupied by blood vessels. These embryonic vessels become unnecessary after the choroid develops, and they are mostly reabsorbed; however, there are often a few remnants of these embryonic vessels floating in the vitreous, and these may be seen from time to time as well. The vitreous possesses scavenger cells (hyalocytes) which assist in removal of debris (such as remnants of old blood vessels, blood cells, or inflammatory cells) from the vitreous. The strongest attachment of the vitreous is to the ciliary body. Next strongest is a ring attachment around the nerve head: when the vitreous detaches, you may see a ring, caused by the shadow of this attachment. There is another, weaker ring attachment around the fovea. In addition, the vitreous has still weaker attachments in the form of strands of collagen anchored to the internal limiting membrane, extending over the entire retinal surface (see Figure 145). When the vitreous condenses with age, any of these attachments may cause traction on the retina, causing the appearance of flashing lights (photopsia) and floaters. In most cases, these symptoms are not significant; however, patients experiencing these symptoms should be examined to rule out more worrisome causes such as retinal detachment.

## SCLERA

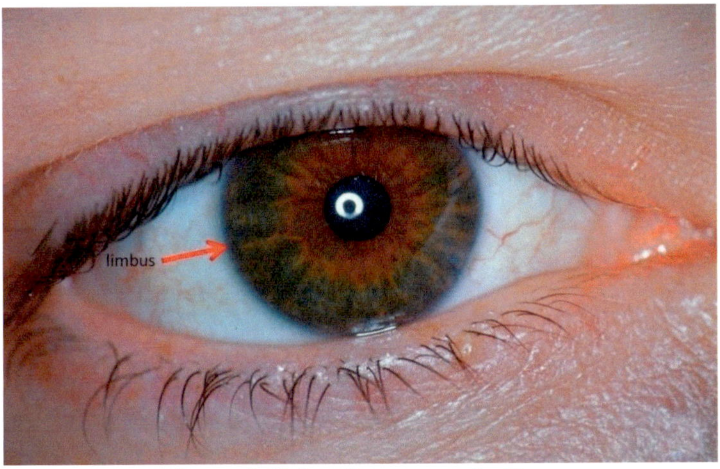


**Figure 9  Join of cornea and sclera**

The white sclera is actually continuous with the cornea. The visible border where cornea ends and sclera begins is called the limbus. The sclera is also continuous with the outermost covering of the brain (the dura mater). The words 'dura' and 'sclera' indicate the layers are quite tough: the cornea is equally tough. At the Optic Nerve Head, there is a sieve-like basketwork of openings in the sclera (the lamina cribrosa) to allow the Ganglion Cell Axons to pass through the sclera into the optic nerve. If there is some depth to the cupping of the nerve head, the white basketwork may be seen, with dark bundles of axons within it (Figure 24). The sclera at the rear of the eye is 1 millimeter thick. The sclera is white and reflects light very strongly. On top of the sclera is a glassy, thin membrane called the conjunctiva. If blood levels of bilirubin (a yellow pigment) are higher than normal (as for example in liver disease), this pigment may accumulate in the conjunctiva. The highly-reflective sclera will show this up and there will be a yellowish appearance to the eye referred to as jaundice.

## CHOROID

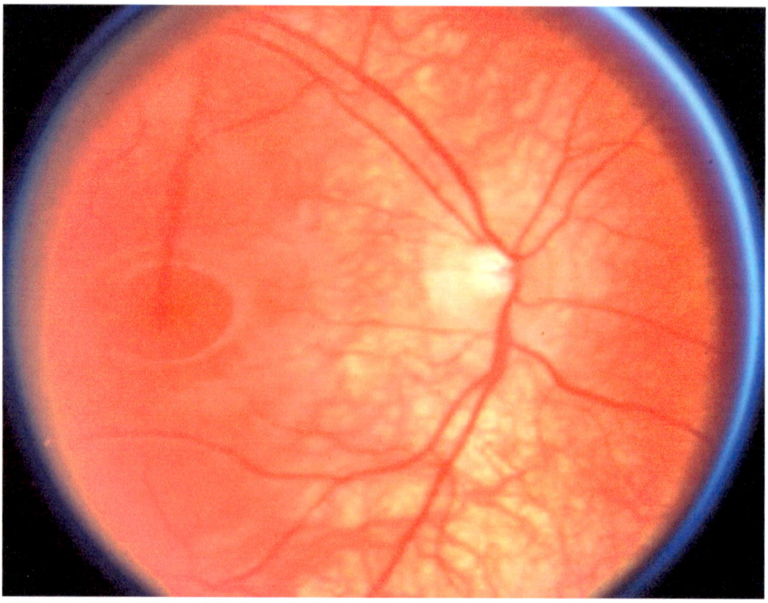

**Figure 10 Choroid visible in person with little RPE pigmentation**

The choroid is a highly vascular layer as it has the job, along with the central retinal circulation, of nourishing the energy-hungry retina. Like all brain tissue, the retina has a high metabolic rate. This person has little pigment in the skin and hair, so there is less pigment in the retinal pigment layer. This allows a view of the feathery, salmon-colored choroidal blood vessels. (When there is more pigmentation of the retinal pigment epithelium, it screens the view of the choroidal vessels.) In the foveal center, the choroid is the sole blood supply of the photoreceptors. The rest of the retina is nourished by both choroid and central retinal circulation. The ciliary body and iris at the front of the eye are part of the choroid (see Figure 1). The circular muscle of the ciliary body controls the shape of the lens, and is represented by black dots, adjacent to the lens in Figure 1. The ciliary body also needs a good blood supply to support its constant production of aqueous humor. At the back of the eye, the choroid is the primary blood supply for the nerve head. The choroid is about 275 micrometers thick and is continuous with the pia mater, the vascular layer on the outside of the optic nerve and the inner side of the brain.

## RETINA

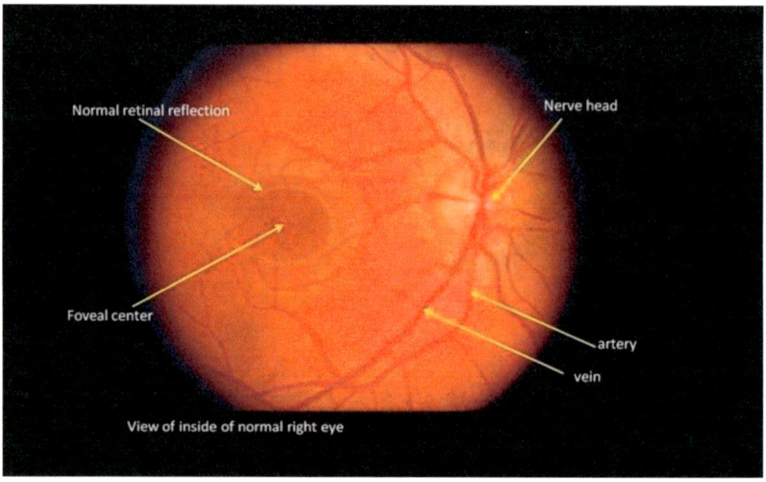


**Figure 11 Retinal circulation, location of foveal center**

The red appearance of this image is because of the blood circulating within and below the transparent retina. The retina is the innermost layer of the eye, and has two parts: the **neuroretina** and the **retinal pigment epithelium** (RPE). The neuroretina contains the photoreceptors (100 million rods and 5 million cones) and their neural connections. The retinal pigment epithelium lies beneath the neuroretina. The vascular layer under the retina is the **choroid**. Separating the retinal pigment epithelium from the choroid is the elastic layer of Bruch (Bruch membrane).

The surface area of the neuroretina is about 1100 square millimeters (about the size of two postage stamps). In most places its thickness is around 200 micrometers (a piece of paper). Light must pass through most of the neuroretina before it reaches the photoreceptors, which rest on the pigment layer (RPE).

A million **Ganglion Cell Axons** from the retina carry information relayed from the receptors by the bipolar cells and ganglion cells. The Ganglion Cell Axons gather together at the nerve head to form the optic nerve, passing through an opening 1.5 millimeters in diameter (about the size of the head of a pin).

Passing through the thickness of the retina are structural cells (**Mueller cells**) which help to bind the retina together. The Mueller cells produce the **internal limiting membrane** of the retina (which faces the vitreous) and the **external limiting membrane** (which faces the retinal pigment epithelium). See Figure 145 for details.
The fovea is a specialized area of the retina: it has only cone photoreceptors present, at the highest density in the whole retina. The rest of the retina has a mixture of rod and cone photoreceptors.

The words 'fovea' and 'macula' are somewhat interchangeable; however, the term 'fovea' has a clear anatomical meaning, so that one is preferable: it is the space between the two thickest parts of the retina (see Figure 168). The size of the fovea is roughly the same as the Optic Nerve Head. The capillary layers of the retinal circulation are absent in the fovea, because they would reduce the sharpness of vision: this means that the fovea has only one blood supply (the choroid). When you look directly at something, the eye turns so that the image falls directly on the foveal center. When you look at stars at night, the fovea is nearly blind, because the cones are not as light-sensitive as the rods. You will have a better chance of seeing a particular star if you look to one side of it, allowing the rods to make a contribution.

As it approaches the ciliary body, the retina thins and rods and cones and their neural connections disappear. The much-thinned retina continues over the ciliary body and the rear surface of the iris, and may usually be seen peeking around the edge of the pupil as the pupillary frill. The retinal pigment epithelium also passes forward over the ciliary body and onto the iris.

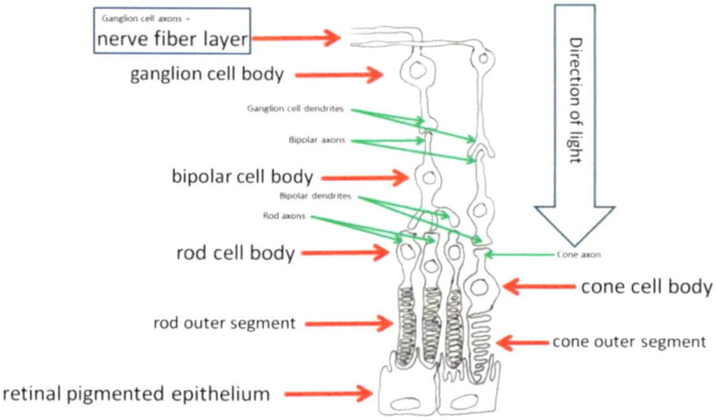


Figure 12 Cells of retina, showing connections

## How do the parts function together?

Light travels through the transparent neuroretina before reaching the photoreceptors (the rods and cones). When photopigment in the receptor outer segments is struck by light, nerve impulses are initiated and travel in a direction opposite to the direction of incoming light as they travel via bipolar cells and ganglion cells to the ganglion cell axons. Look at the edge of a piece of paper: all these retinal layers are inside its thickness (~200 micrometers).

Impulses in nerves usually travel from the dendrite toward the axon. Where an axon is in contact with the dendrite of the next neuron in the pathway is called a synapse: two synapses are shown in this figure.

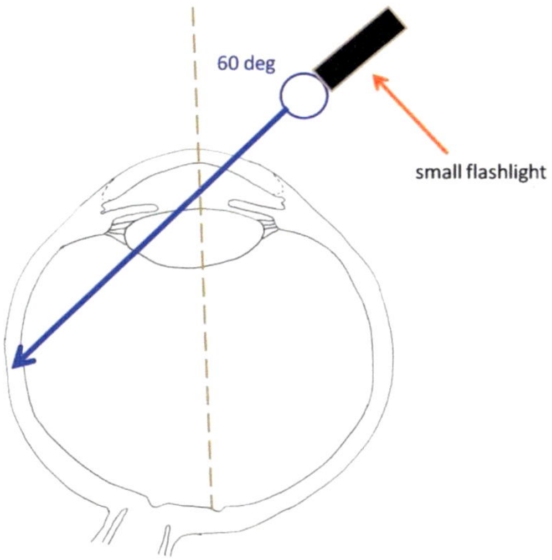


**Figure 13 How to see Purkinje tree**

The third synapse in the visual pathway is at the lateral geniculate body, where the Ganglion Cell Axons contact the dendrites of the optic radiation fibers. The fibers of the optic radiations carry the impulses the rest of the way to the visual cortex. Simpler organisms have light receptors closer to the light. See Figure 37 for some explanation of the 'upside-down' orientation of the human photoreceptors.

Some ganglion cells possess a photopigment (melanopsin) which allows them to respond to light in the 481 nanometer range. These cells respond to overall light level, and are thought to help establish circadian rhythms. Opsins in one form or another are found in many living things, from fruit flies to fish to humans.

Occasionally, when light is directed obliquely into the eye, you can see shadows of the blood vessels of the retinal circulation. These blood vessels do lie on top of the photoreceptors of the eye, and you might reasonably expect to see shadows of these blood vessels all the time. The visual system has made several adaptations to avoid this. The visual system is more interested in things that change than in things which stay still, so unchanging shadows tend to be ignored.

There is another thing the eye does to avoid seeing the same thing all the time: the eye constantly shows a very slight movement (micronystagmus), which has the effect of constantly refreshing the photoreceptors.

Here is a sketch of what you might see when the flashlight is directed into the right eye as shown in Figure 13. This appearance is made more visible by slightly wiggling the flashlight, either in a horizontal or vertical direction. You will notice that there is a small area which is avoided by the blood vessel shadows: this is the foveal center. The larger blood vessel shadows you see are originating at the right side of the picture, because these blood vessels enter and leave the eye at the nerve head.

The actual entrance and exit of the main blood vessels will not be seen, as this corresponds with the blind spot. The blind spot for the right eye lies to the right of the straight-ahead position. By directing the light into the eye obliquely, you are overcoming the mechanisms which usually make these shadows invisible. The tree-like appearance was described in 1823 by Purkinje, who also did extensive research on the neurons of the brain.

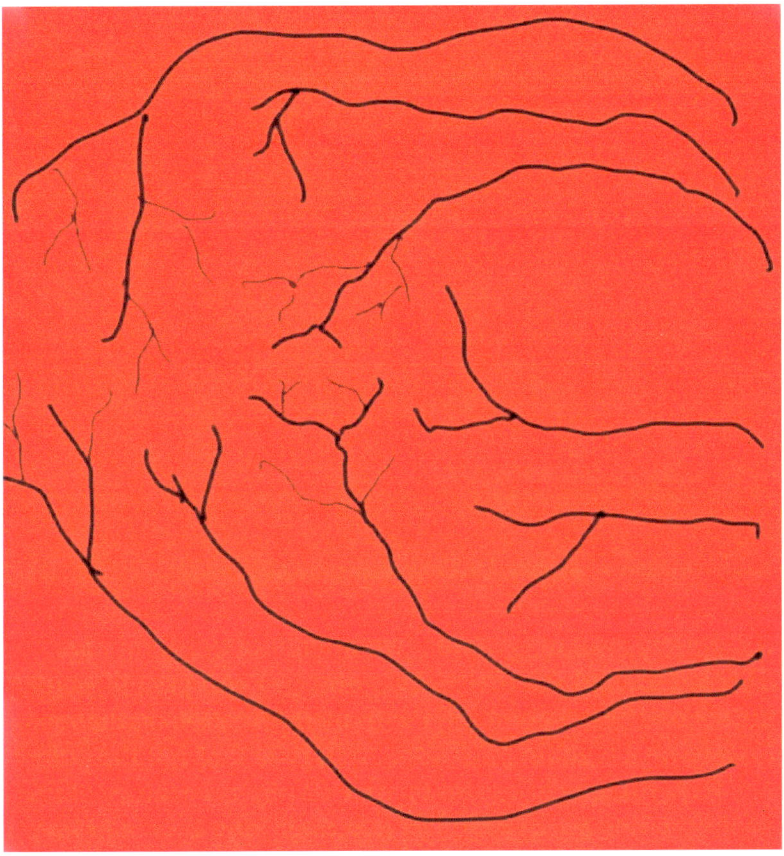

**Figure 14 Sketch of the Purkinje tree**

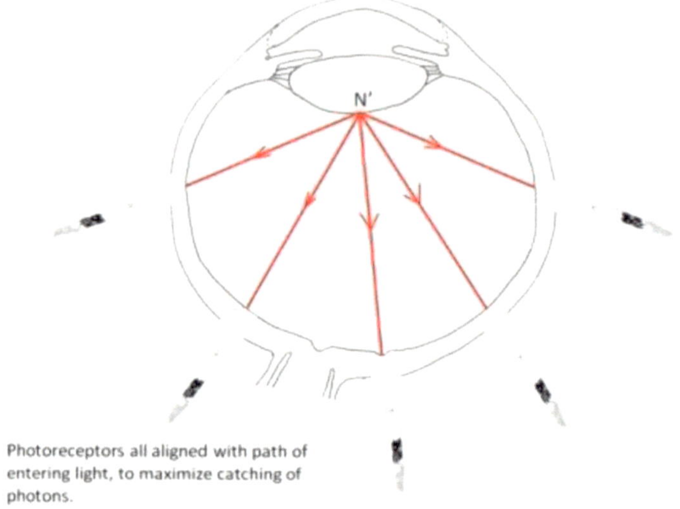


**Figure 15 Photoreceptor alignment**

All optical systems possess two nodal points: light rays directed toward the first nodal point (N) will pass through the second nodal point (N') with their direction unchanged. So any rays reaching the retina will pass through the point N'. Experiments have shown that all photoreceptors of the healthy retina are oriented so that their long axis is in line with light rays which pass through the second nodal point, N'. The photoreceptors also have their photopigment (in their outer segment) oriented at right angles to their long axis. These two orientations so effectively maximize the chance to catch photons that a single photon is capable of triggering the visual process.

The alignment of the photoreceptor axes is disturbed following a retinal detachment; however, in the months following correction of a retinal detachment, millions of photoreceptors use their mobility to return to their original alignment.

Figure 16 is a sketch of the entire retina of a right eye as it would be seen when you are looking directly at the patient. The yellowish horizontal v-shaped areas are places where major nerves and long posterior ciliary blood vessels are running in the space between the choroid and the sclera. The feathery patterns converging at points are veins of the choroid, the middle, vascular layer of the eye. The small white circle at the center is the Optic Nerve Head, and the cross temporal to the nerve head marks the foveal center.

The retina may be described as having four quadrants, based on imaginary lines passing horizontally and vertically through the nerve head: thus, there are superior and inferior nasal quadrants and superior and inferior temporal quadrants. A different organization is used when describing the visual field, where the fovea is the central point.

When an eye care practitioner examines the retina with a conventional ophthalmoscope, the view is limited to one or two nerve head diameters. With other instruments, such as the indirect ophthalmoscope, the view is larger, as in Fig. 11. With other instruments, the retina may be seen all the way to its edges, where the serrations are seen, particularly on the nasal side, but only portions of the peripheral retina may be seen at any one time.

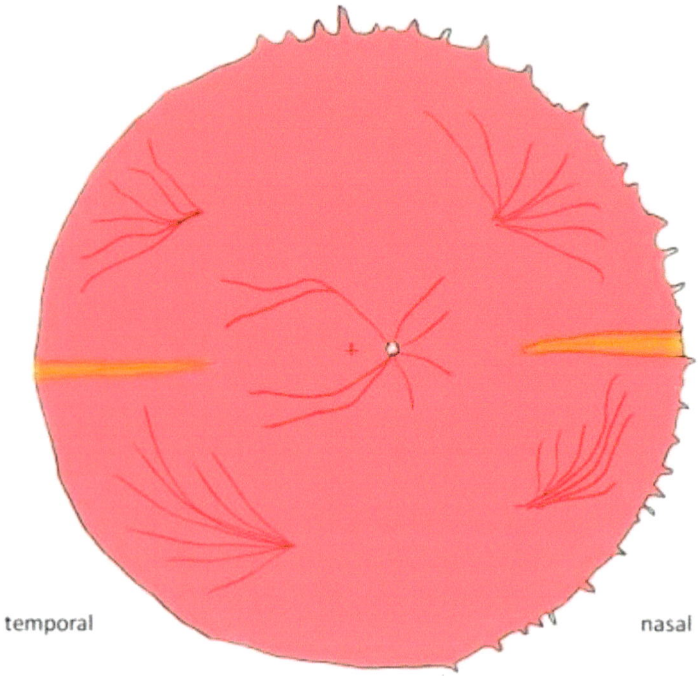


Figure 16  Sketch of whole retina

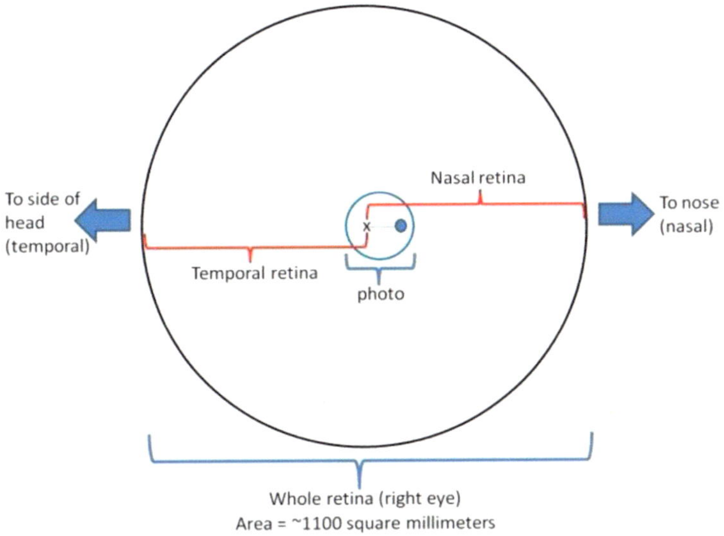


**Figure 17  Divisions of retina**

The whole retina was sketched in the Figure 16. Here is a reminder that only a small portion of the retina may be seen at a time in fine detail. The surface area of the whole retina is approximately 1100 square millimeters, while the area seen in conventional photos like Fig. 11 is more like 65 square millimeters. The foveal center (marked with an 'X') is shown at the center of this sketch; the nerve head lies nasal to the foveal center (that is, toward the nose). The foveal center divides the retina into nasal and temporal portions when the visual field is being considered.

# retina: cones

- 5 million
- daytime vision
- color vision
- high resolution
- poor motion detection
- densest at foveal center
- found throughout retina

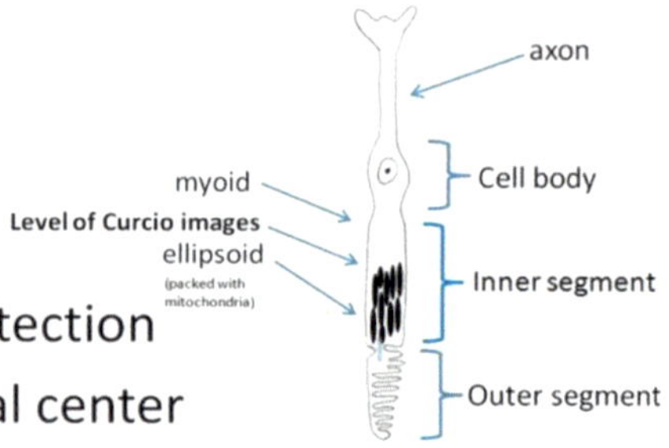


**Figure 18 Cone Details**

The fovea centralis contains cones only. The high density of mitochondria (shown here as black, cigar-shaped objects) in the inner segment of the cone reflects the intense activity of making new photopigment molecules, which are delivered to the outer segment. The diameter of mitochondria is around 1 micrometer. All Cilia possess nine microtubule pairs connecting their inner and outer segments. Mobile cilia have a central tenth pair which makes them capable of movement, like the photoreceptors. Fine lines between the inner and outer segment of photoreceptors represent the ten microtubule pairs, confirming that photoreceptors are modified Cilia. Curcio et al. (J Comp Neurol 1990;292:497-523) obtained images of the cones at the join between the myoid and ellipsoid of the receptor inner segments.

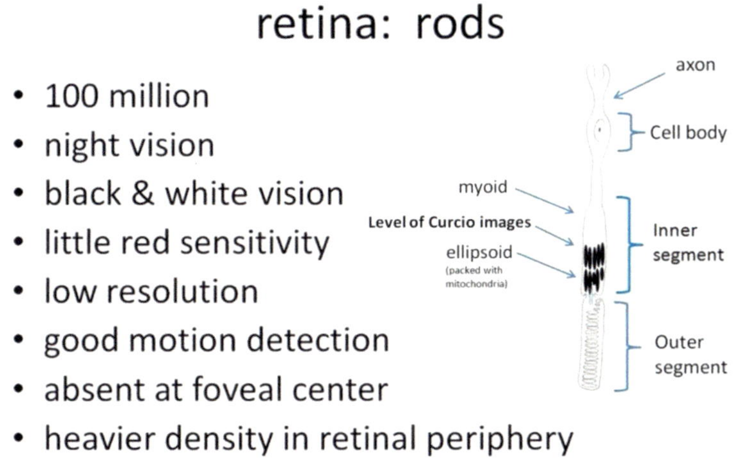


**Figure 19 Rod Details**

Rods are found everywhere in the retina, except for the fovea and the extreme periphery. They are more numerous than cones. Again, fine lines between inner and outer segments represent the ten microtubule pairs which are characteristic of mobile Cilia.

In rods, photopigment is contained in membrane discs of the outer segment; in cones, photopigment is contained within infoldings of the cell membrane. In each case, the layers of photopigment are at right angles to the direction of light travel.

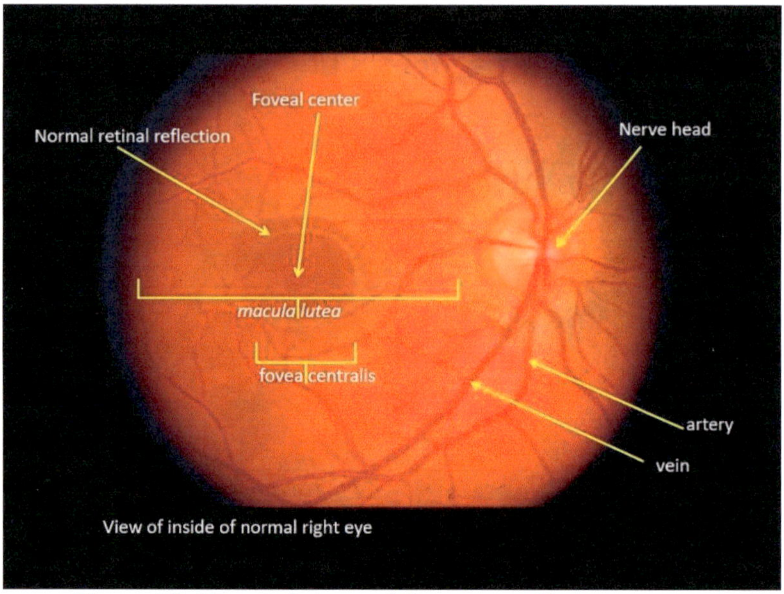


**Figure 20 Macula lutea and fovea centralis**

The macula lutea (Latin for yellow spot) is an ill-defined area surrounding the foveal center. The retina in this area possesses a yellow-absorbing pigment, LUTEIN.

On the other hand, the fovea centralis (Latin for central depression) is perfectly defined by the circular reflection in this retinal photo (marked by the yellow arrow and bracket). This is a reflection from the convex, thickest part of the retina, giving the reflection marked in Figure 20. The thickest part of the retina is 370 micrometers (where the peaks of the fovea centralis are found) and its thinnest part is at the foveal center, where it is 130 micrometers thick. The foveal center contains cones only. All other retinal structures (bipolar cells, ganglion cells, and their neural connections) are displaced from the foveal center, which is why there is such a great thickness at the edges of the fovea centralis. Mueller cells are also displaced to the side, making the macula vulnerable to swelling. Distance from foveal center to nerve head center is usually about 15 degrees (three Optic Nerve Head diameters, about 4.5 millimeters [4500 micrometers]). Usually, the fovea centralis is about the same width as the nerve head. See Figure 168 for more detail on the fovea.

**Amsler Grid**

The Amsler grid is a pattern of squares, each 5 mm on the side. The whole grid is 20 x 20 squares, so it is 10 cm x 10 cm. Viewed at a distance of 28 cm, each 5 mm square is one degree in size.

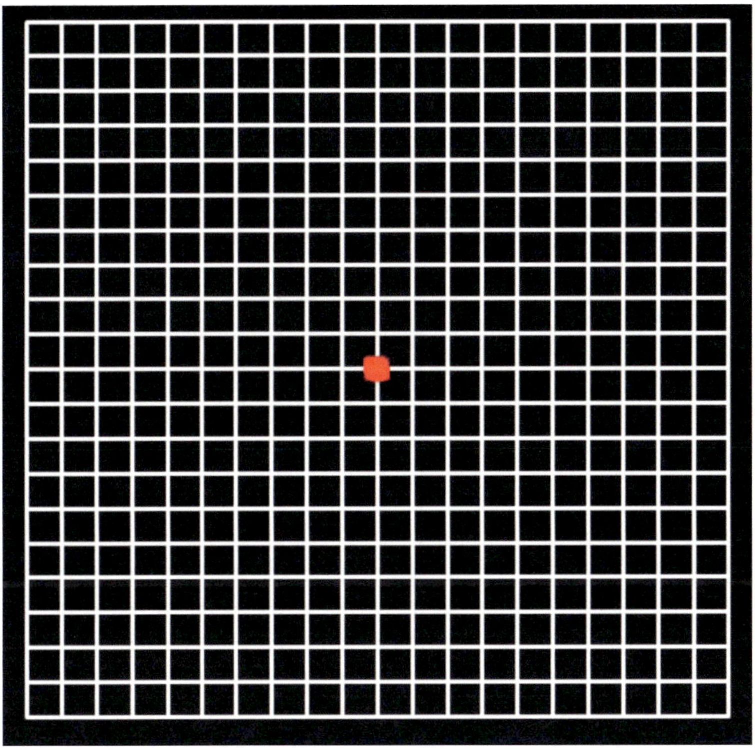

Figure 21 Amsler grid

**Instructions for Patient:**

To use this Amsler grid, wear your reading glasses (if needed), cover one eye, hold the book 28 centimeters (11 inches) from your eye, and look steadily at the red spot at the center of the grid. Can you see all four corners? Can you see all four sides? Are there any missing squares? Do all of the squares actually look square? Make a sketch of any abnormalities and show it to your eye care practitioner.

.

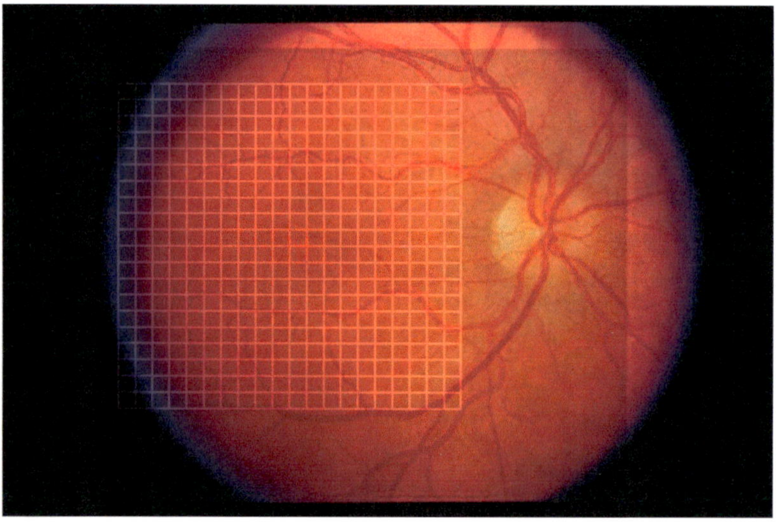

**Figure 22 Amsler grid imaged on retina**

Here we see the Amsler grid imaged to scale on the retina. The patient with (for example) macular degeneration will notice missing areas in the grid. If there were areas of fluid under the retina, this will cause some of the squares to appear smaller than their neighbours. This picture shows why the blindspot is not detected by the Amsler grid.

A crossword puzzle can serve as a reasonable substitute for the Amsler grid.

## OPTIC NERVE HEAD

The Optic Nerve Head (see rectangle below) is the portion of the optic nerve which lies ahead of the lamina cribrosa. Large red arrows show inputs from the choroid into the Optic Nerve Head.

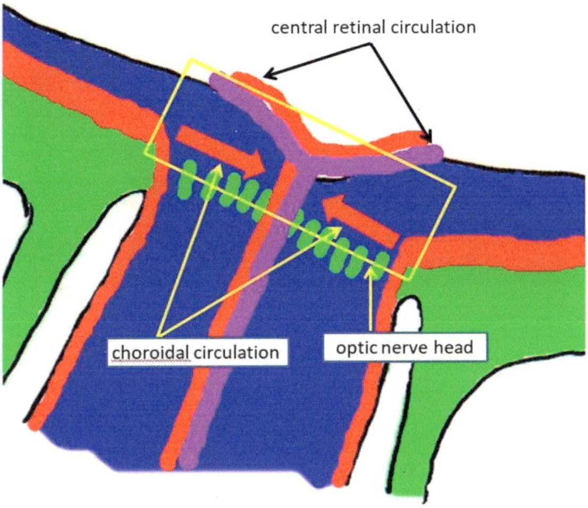


Figure 23 Nerve Head Detail

**The choroid is the chief blood supply of the Optic Nerve Head area**. Half of the optic nerve head is occupied by astroglial cells, which intervene between the blood vessels of the nerve head and the ganglion cell axons and provide various protections for the axons. Raised intraocular pressure (IOP) may collapse some of the choroidal blood vessels nourishing axons in the nerve head. In addition, raised IOP may cause axon damage due to stretching of axons and their related astroglial cells. Affected axons may slowly fail and die. The central retinal artery and vein pass through the Optic Nerve Head on their way to supply the inner retina. Moving away from the eyeball, the optic nerve itself is nourished by the central retinal circulation on the inside of the nerve, and the pia mater on the outside of the nerve. There are no rods or cones at the Optic Nerve Head, which is why everyone has a blind spot.

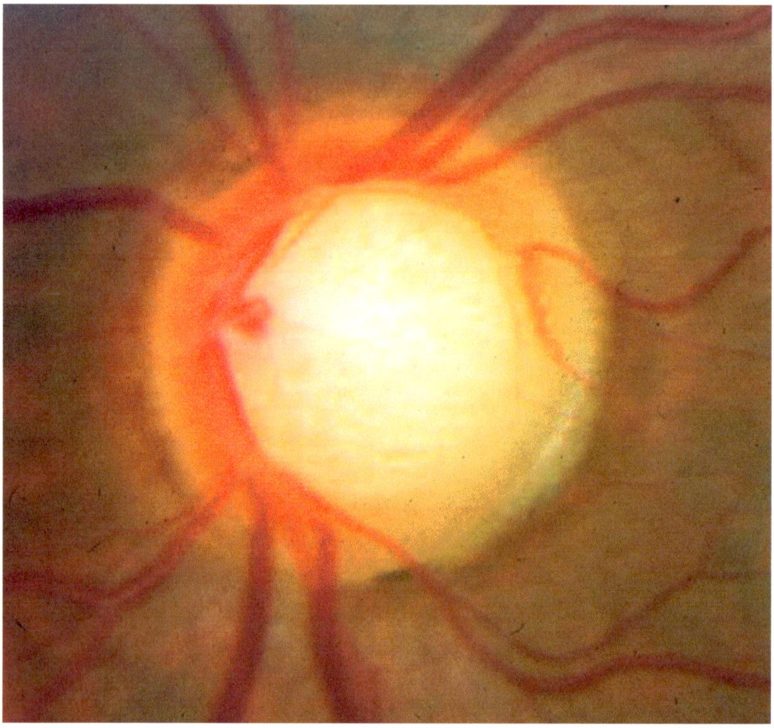

**Figure 24 Optic Nerve Head**

Here is a close up of a healthy left Optic Nerve Head with a relatively wide and deep cupping. The configuration of the nerve head varies greatly among individuals, but is usually similar from one eye to the other. In the bottom of the cupping, faint grayish polygons may be seen: these are bundles of ganglion cell axons leaving the eye. The whitish basketwork between the grayish polygons is the lamina cribrosa. For nerve heads with little or no cupping, the lamina cribrosa is not visible. The retinal pigment epithelium halts at the margin of the optic nerve head. The opening in the sclera is 1.5 millimeters wide. It is amazing that one million retinal ganglion cell axons pass through it to form the optic nerve.

**This is a demonstration of the blind spot for your left eye.**

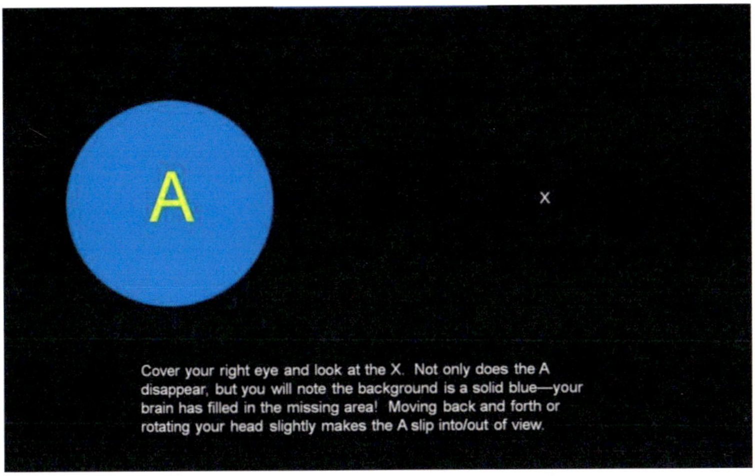


Figure 25 Demonstration of Blind Spot

Close your right eye and hold your book 8.8 inches (22 cm) away from your eye, a bit closer than your usual reading distance. For the blind spot of your right eye, turn your book 180 degrees.

Most people are surprised to learn they have a blind spot, but there it is. For people with longer than average eyeballs (say longer than 22 millimeters), the blindspot will be somewhat larger and moved outward, and the reverse is true for shorter eyeballs. For people with two normal eyes, the blindspots are of no practical significance, because the vision of each eye compensates for the blind spot of the other eye.

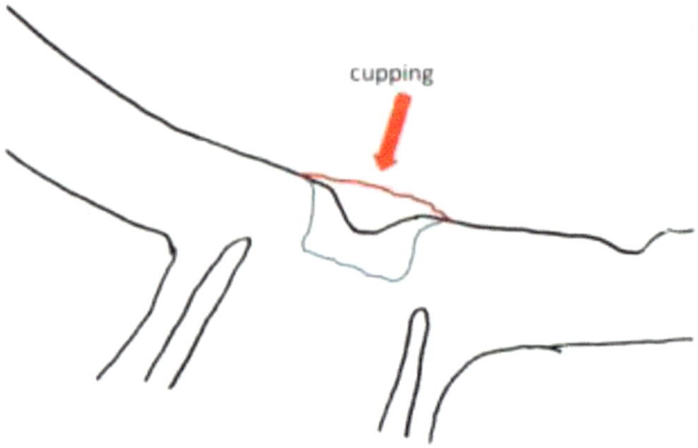


Figure 26 Different cuppings

At the center of the Optic Nerve Head there is usually an indentation, called the cupping. There are many variations in the normal eye (Figure 26). As shown in red, the eye may have no cupping at all, and the nerve head may even look slightly convex; in other cases, there may be a small depression (shown in black). In still other normal cases, there may be a deeper cupping (shown in blue). The cupping in the last case may be a millimeter or more deep. Of concern in cases of glaucoma is a progressive deepening and widening of the cupping, which indicates loss of Ganglion Cell Axons.

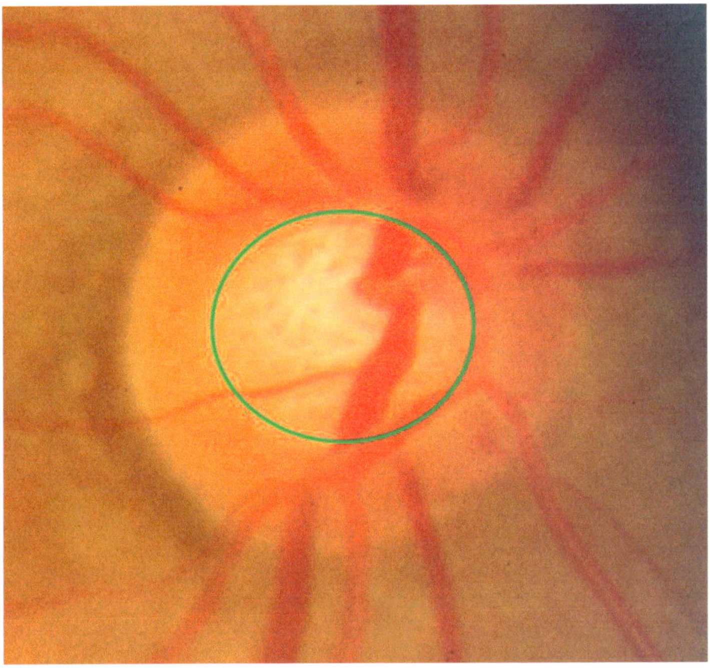

Figure 27 Locating edge of cupping

Both the retinal pigment epithelium and photoreceptor layers end at the edges of the optic nerve head. The darker pigmentation of the retinal pigment epithelium halts at the edge of the nerve head. This right nerve head has a cupping like that shown in blue in Figure 26. At the nerve head, the transparent Ganglion Cell Axons turn downward (away from the eye) to enter the optic nerve. The width of the cupping in the nerve head is shown approximately by the green ellipse in Figure 27. The trunk of the central retinal vein is visible in the floor of the cupping. It is invariably temporal to the central retinal artery trunk. The gray polygons in the floor of the cupping are bundles of Ganglion Cell Axons passing through the white meshwork of the lamina cribrosa. These features are visible because of the depth of the cupping. Part of the assessment of a nerve head is to measure how deep and wide the cupping is.

## OPTIC NERVE

The optic nerve is a cranial nerve and is also known as the second of the twelve cranial nerves. The optic nerve is covered by the meninges of the brain (pia mater, Arachnoid, and dura mater, as shown in Figure 29). Once the ganglion cell axons pass the lamina cribrosa, they continue along the optic nerve, through the chiasm, and end at the lateral geniculate body in the midbrain, where they connect with the final neurons (the optic radiations) which go to the visual cortex at the back of the head.

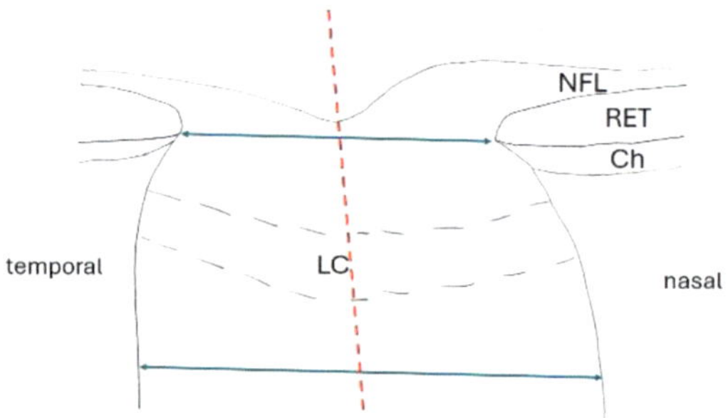


Figure 28 optic nerve size

Both the retina (ret) and choroid (Ch) halt at the edge of the optic nerve head. Once the million Ganglion Cell Axons (NFL) from the retina pass through the multiple openings in the sclera (the lamina cribrosa LC), they make up the optic nerve.

The optic nerve is not readily observed in a routine eye examination. The opening through which the visual nerve fibers pass is only 1.5 mm wide (about the size of the head of a pin). Further back, the optic nerve is thicker than you might expect, because the fibers are heavily insulated with myelin (produced by oligodendrocytes of the central nervous system) once they are behind the lamina cribrosa. Myelin on the Ganglion Cell Axons while they are in the retina would interfere with vision.

The dashed red line in Figure 28 shows the direction of the optic nerve. This direction may vary from person to person but is usually similar in an individual. The optic nerve orientation shown in Figure 28 is typical of a myopic eye: often the greater the degree of myopia, the greater the angling toward the nasal side.

Peripheral nerves have their myelin produced by Schwann cells outside the central nervous system, and are capable of regeneration, while central nerves like the optic nerve are not capable of regeneration.

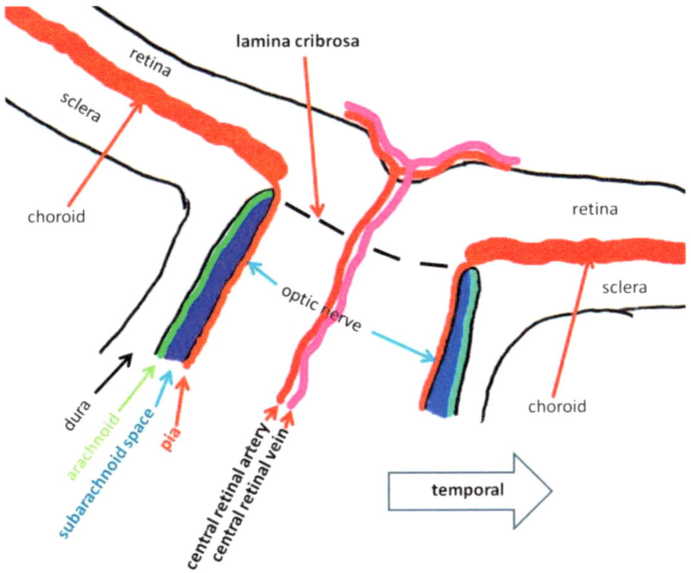


Figure 29 Coverings of Optic Nerve

The three coverings of the brain surround the optic nerve. The white, outer covering of the eye (sclera) is continuous with the outer covering of the brain (dura mater). The vascular layer closest to the nerve is the pia mater. Outside that is the subarachnoid space, and outside that are the Arachnoid and the dura layers. These three layers (collectively called the meninges) cover the entire optic nerve, brain and spinal cord. Just as the eye is filled with aqueous humor, the ventricles of the brain and the subarachnoid space are filled with cerebrospinal fluid. The pia mater is connected to the choroid, which lies under the retina. The subarachnoid space comes almost to the eyeball, halting at the lamina cribrosa. Raised pressure in the subarachnoid space can cause compression of the optic nerve and also the vessels of the central retinal circulation.

The central retinal artery and vein travel within the optic nerve, passing through the lamina cribrosa to enter the eye. The central retinal vein is always temporal to the central retinal artery and leaves the optic nerve about 10 millimeters behind the globe, to drain into the brain's venous system. The central retinal artery enters the optic nerve also about 10 millimeters behind the globe.

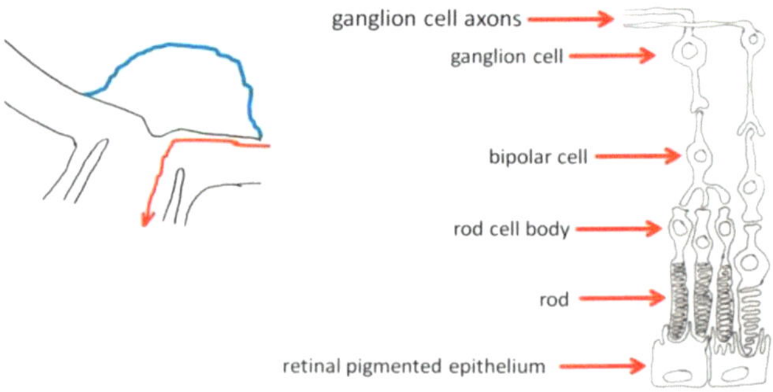


Figure 30  Nerve Head in papilledema

The retinal Ganglion Cell Axons are not just wires. The microtubules of axons are responsible for transport of various materials (for example proteins and neurotransmitters) in both directions along the axon. The movement of materials away from the ganglion cell body is called **orthograde** axoplasmic flow, while movement toward the ganglion cell body is called **retrograde** axoplasmic flow. The red arrow on the left part of Figure 30 shows not only the path of the axons but also the orthograde path of axoplasmic transport.

Axoplasmic flow transports factors needed for the health of the nerve as well as chemicals necessary for transmission of nerve impulses. It is a mechanism by which all nerves in a pathway stay in touch with each other: damage to one nerve in the pathway ultimately leads to damage to all connected nerves in the pathway. If the optic nerve fibers are compressed due to increased pressure in the subarachnoid space, then axoplasmic material from the ganglion cell body accumulates in the nerve head and causes swelling (papilledema). Hemorrhages or tumors within the brain may cause papilledema. Severe hypertension may cause it also. The surface of the nerve head may rise by 2-3 millimeters (shown in blue) in some cases.

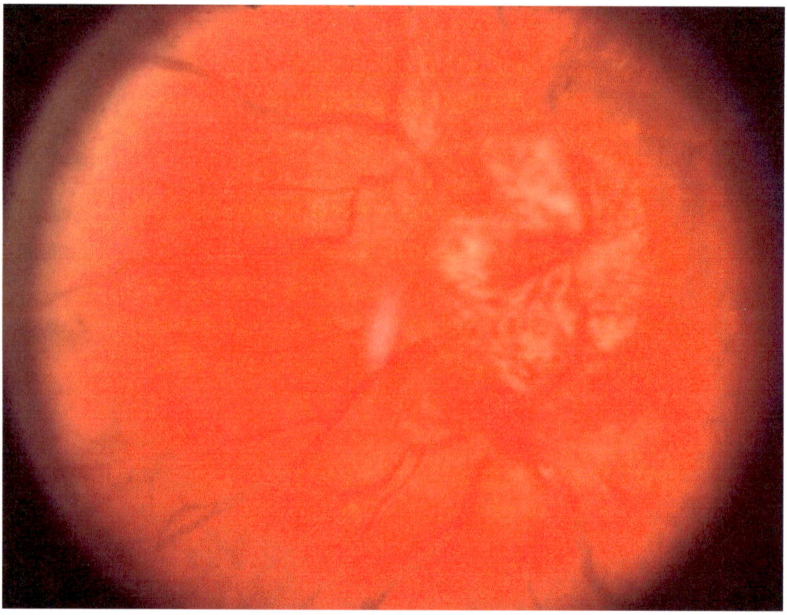

Figure 31 Clinical view of papilledema

Here is an example of papilledema. The swelling of the nerve head has made its borders very indistinct, and the blood vessels at the center of the nerve head are blurred because they are elevated to a point a millimetre or more higher than the adjacent retina level. The swelling occurred because raised intracranial pressure squeezed the axons travelling through the optic nerve, preventing the orthograde flow of materials toward the end of the axon in the midbrain: these materials accumulated on the retinal side of the optic nerve. Because there are no Mueller fibers in the nerve head to hold the retina together, dramatic swelling may develop

# Chapter 2 EMBRYONIC DEVELOPMENT OF THE EYE

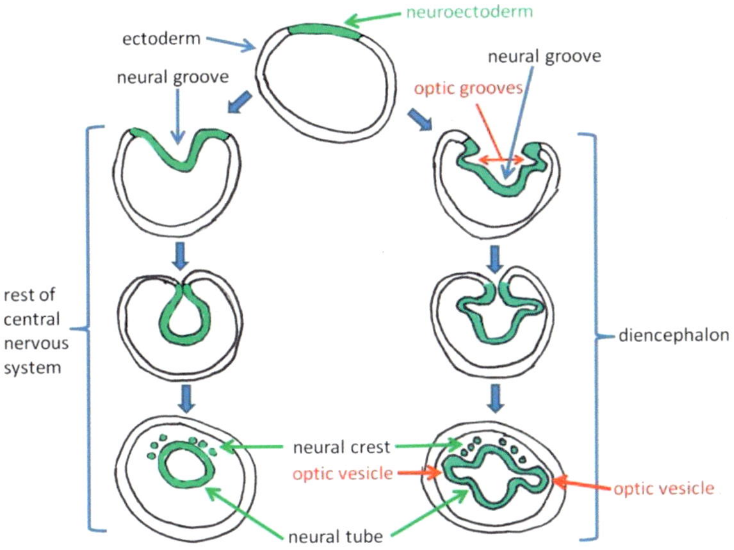


Figure 32 Appearance of optic vesicle

The embryo has three layers which give rise to the following:

- ectoderm (central and peripheral nervous systems, all pigment cells [except for the retinal pigment epithelium], the corneal epitheium, lens of the eye, skin, hair, and tooth enamel);
- mesoderm (circulatory system, skeleton, and muscles); and
- endoderm (digestive and respiratory systems).

Ectoderm gives rise **to surface ectoderm** (white) and **neuroectoderm** (green) in Figure 32.

Neuroectoderm folds in and separates from the surface ectoderm. About 28 days after conception, the neural tube forms along the length of the embryo. When the edges of the infolding neuroectoderm fuse, some cells remain between the neural tube and the surface ectoderm. These cells are called the neural crest. In the forebrain's diencephalon portion, the infolding neuroectoderm has additional infoldings called the optic grooves. When the neural tube separates from the surface ectoderm, these grooves enlarge to form the optic vesicles.

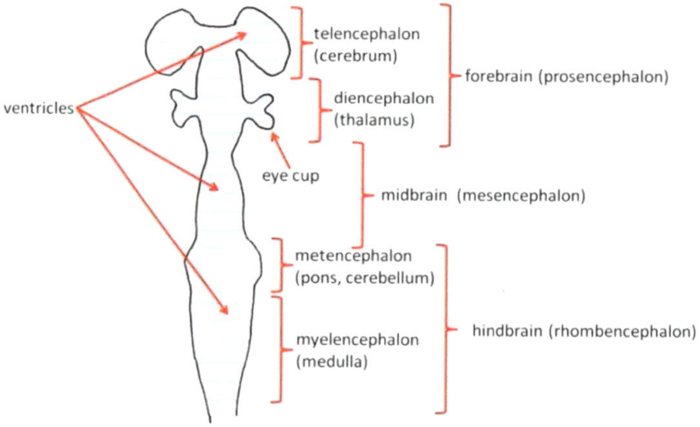


**Figure 33 Embryonic brain**

The brain of the embryo 29 days after conception is a hollow tube. The eye develops from part of the forebrain in the form first of a bulge (the optic vesicle), which then folds in on itself to form the optic cup, also known as the eye cup. The future retinal pigment epithelium is beginning to show some pigmentation by 35 days after conception.

Here is a look at the developing nervous system of a 36-day human embryo. The neural tube has closed and moved within the embryo, and is shown in red. The future brain occupies much of the head end of the embryo. By this stage, the outer part of the eye cup (the future retinal pigment epithelium) has started to become pigmented, and may be seen through the translucent surface of the embryo.

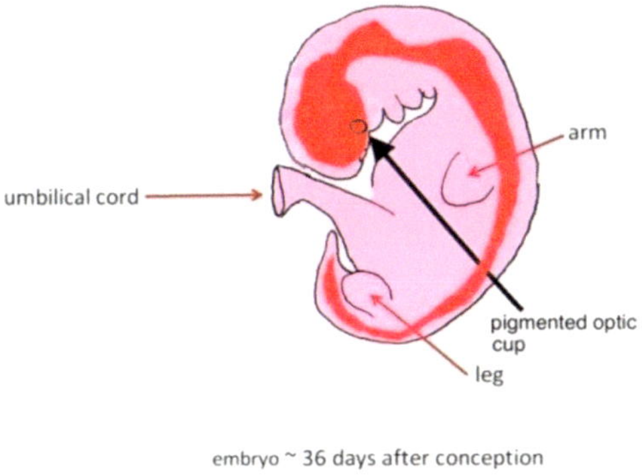


**Figure 34 Brain within embryo**

The early development of the human visual system resembles that of fish: in fish and humans, the eyes first appear on the sides of the head. In the fish, the eyes remain on the side of the head, and most of the Ganglion Cell Axons cross over to the other side of the brain. In humans, the eyes migrate toward the front of the head. In humans, the nasal retina and its crossing Ganglion Cell Axons develop about <u>30 days</u> before the non-crossing axons from the temporal retina, a reminder of our fishy ancestors. Having non-crossing axons makes binocular vision possible. Generally speaking, the more frontal the position of the eyes, the greater the percentage of non-crossing temporal axons.

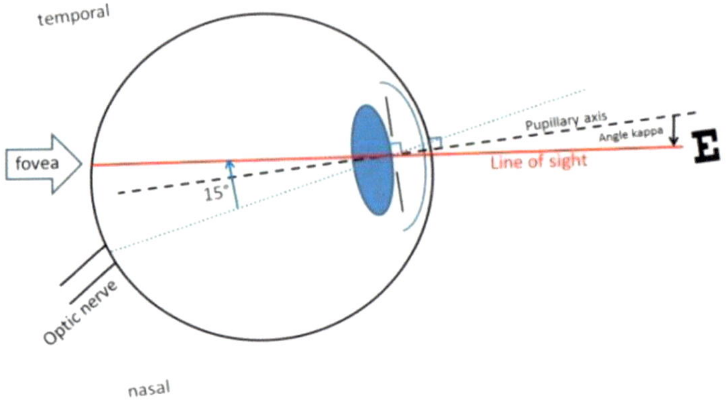


Figure 35  Angle kappa detail

This is a left eye, as viewed from above. This eye is looking straight ahead: the line of sight connects the fovea with the object you are looking at (the letter 'E' in this case). The rest of the optical system of the eye (cornea and lens) has its axis (known as the pupillary or optical axis) lined up somewhat toward the left of what you are looking at. In the embryo, with the eyes on the sides of the head, the pupillary axes are nearly ninety degrees away from their final position. The adult eye shows a small, lingering sign of the old, 'side-looking' alignment. The discrepancy between line of sight and pupillary (or optical) axis, the angle kappa, is on average 5 degrees, as though the pupillary axis is trying to catch up with the new line of sight. The Optic Nerve Head is on average 15 degrees from the line of sight.

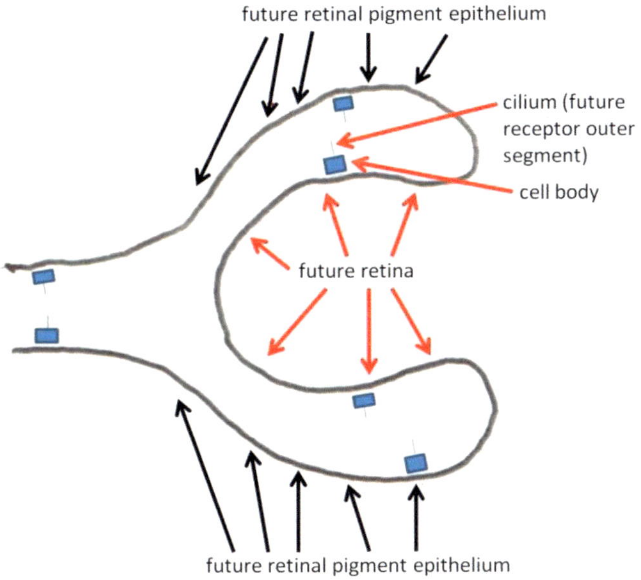


**Figure 36 Ependymal cells**

The central nervous system is completely lined by ependymal cells with hair-like Cilia (singular cilium). A few ependymal cells are represented here as blue rectangles with little hairs (Cilia) attached. Cilia are connected to the cell body by ten pairs of fine filaments which move the Cilia. Within the ventricles of the brain and spinal cord, these Cilia move the cerebrospinal fluid around. When the optic vesicle bulges out from the forebrain during embryonic development, it brings ependymal cells with it.

When the retina develops, the Cilia of these cells are modified to become the light-sensitive outer segments of rods and cones, which gives an explanation for the apparent ‘upside down’ order of cells in the retina.

In other organisms such as the single-celled ***Euglena viridans***, light receptors are found close to the body surface: light hits the light-sensitive receptor first and then the receptor body passes information to the flagellum, which moves the organism to the best position for receiving light. In the human retina, light has to pass through the cell body of the receptor BEFORE it reaches the light-sensitive part of the receptor. In other words, the nerve impulses in the human retina travel OPPOSITE to the direction of light. The Cilia of the future retinal pigment epithelial cells do not develop into receptor outer segments, but instead the Cilia of the retinal pigment epithelial cells are wrapped around the photoreceptor outer segments.

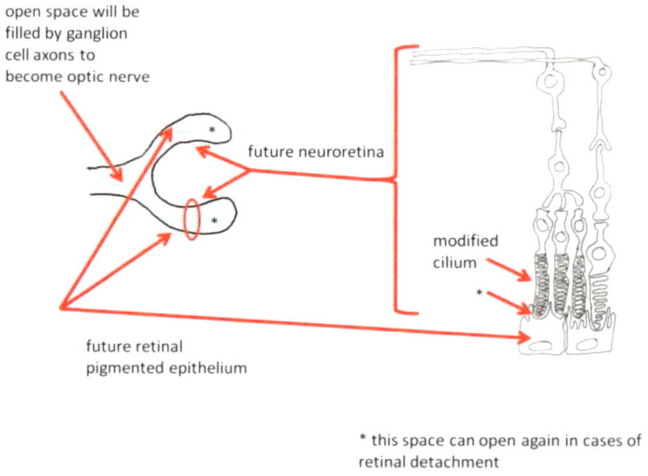


**Figure 37 Origins of neuroretina and RPE**

There are three different areas of pigment to discuss:

- Pigment at the bottom of the retina (the retinal pigment epithelium)
- Pigment in the iris
- Pigment in the rods and cones (the photoreceptors)

# RETINAL PIGMENT EPITHELIUM (RPE)

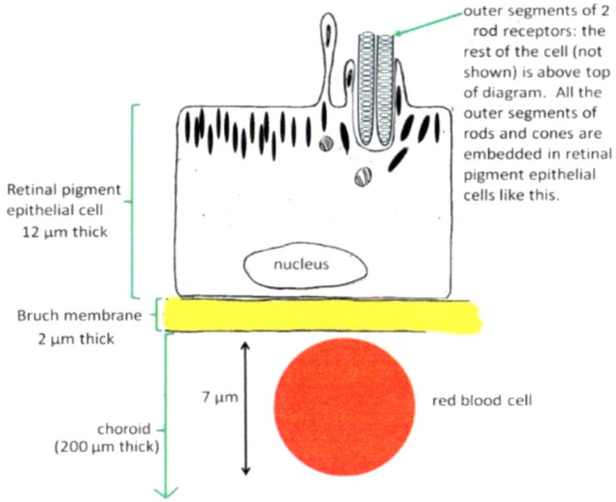


Figure 38 RPE, Bruch membrane, choroid

RPE comes from the embryonic optic cup, and is the only pigmented cell in the whole body which comes from **NEUROECTODERM.** The RPE nourishes photoreceptor outer segments and provides to their inner segments the necessary materials to replace photopigment. The RPE pumps fluid constantly out of the space between itself and the receptor outer segments; otherwise the neural part of the retina would detach. In addition, the RPE scavenges shed photoreceptor material at night, when it becomes exhausted. RPE cells have a range of responses, varying from pigment loss when damage is slight (Fig. 169) to proliferation when they are strongly stimulated (Fig. 149).

The pigment contained by RPE cells is melanin, which is also contained by all the pigment cells of the rest of the body (the MELANOCYTES). The melanocytes are derived from the **NEURAL CREST**. The amount of melanin found in the iris, skin, hair, and RPE is similar: people with dark eyes, hair and skin have lots of melanin in their RPE cells, while people with blue eyes, light hair and skin have much less melanin in their RPE.

The asterisks in the left of Figure 37 mark the original subretinal space in the embryo, while the single asterisk on the right marks what is left of the subretinal space in the fully-developed retina. The subretinal space which used to exist between these two layers during embryonic development may appear again between the receptor outer segments and the RPE in cases of retinal detachment. The circled area matches the orientation of the finally-developed retina and RPE shown on the right. The modified cilia labelled in the diagram are the receptor outer segments. Photopigment is in them.

## PIGMENT IN THE IRIS

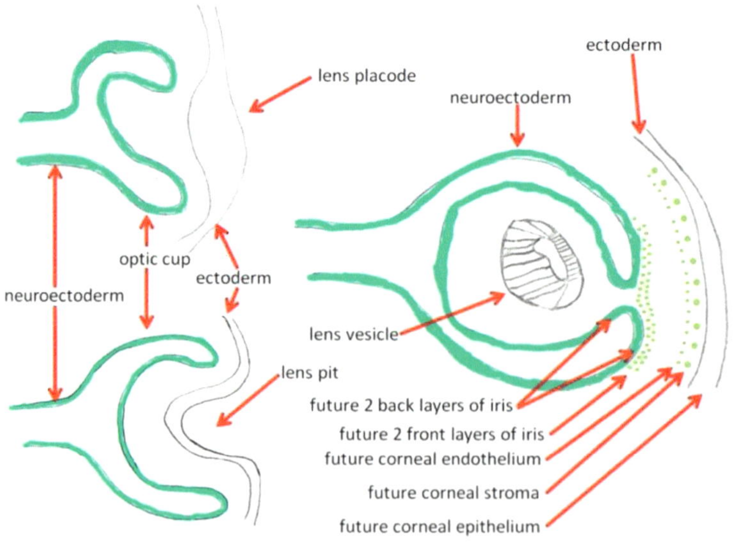


Figure 39 Embryo iris, cornea, lens

The two layers at the front of the optic cup wind up as the two back pigment layers of the iris; the more posterior pigment layer is derived from the retina and the more anterior pigment layer from the retinal pigment epithelium. These two pigment layers are very good at blocking light from passing through the iris. In the lighter green dots, you will see that the neural crest supplies the corneal stroma, corneal endothelium, and 2 layers on the very front of the iris. In the embryo, the very front layer goes across the pupil (the pupillary membrane); however, before birth it withers away back to the location of the future collarette. Sometimes in the fully-formed eye there is a vestige of this pupillary membrane, which looks like a fine cobweb in the anterior chamber (Figure 40). It has no impact on vision, in most cases. The corneal epithelium comes from the surface ectoderm.

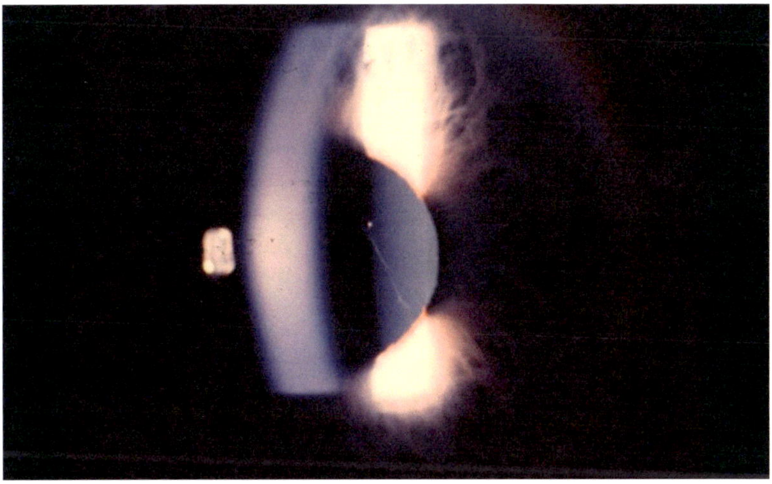

**Figure 40 Persistent pupillary membrane**

The rest of the iris pigment (which determines eye color) develops later in the front two layers of the iris. The front two layers are not good at stopping passage of light. Blue irises have little melanin, while brown ones have much melanin. At the edge of the pupil in most eyes, a frill of golden brown pigment (the pupillary frill) is visible (see Figure 44): it has actually rolled around from the posterior pigment layer of the iris: so there is a little bit of retinal tissue right out front at the edge of the iris!

## THE CILIARY BODY AND ITS PIGMENT LAYERS

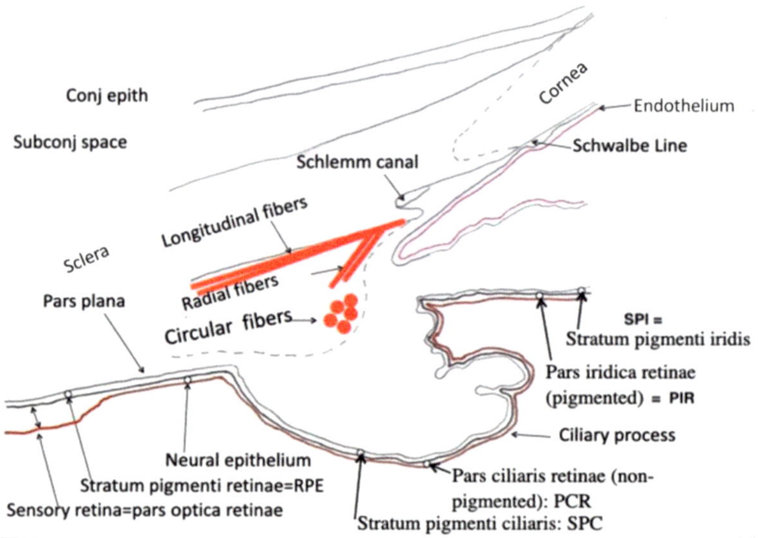


**Figure 41 Pigment layers of retina, ciliary body, iris**

Here is too much detail about the ciliary body region, but it gives an opportunity to understand the two pigment layers on the back of the iris. (A little Latin terminology never hurt anyone!) These two layers come from the optic cup: the pigment layer at the back of the iris (PIR) comes from the inner part of the optic cup, and the pigment layer ahead of that (SPI) comes from the outer part of the optic cup. If you work your way along the bottom of the diagram, you will see the thicker portion of the sensory retina (the pars optica retinae) gradually become thinner as it wraps around the ciliary process, finally becoming the back layer of the iris.

The retinal pigment epithelium (RPE) follows the same course, winding up in front of the retinal part on the back of the iris. The retina itself is transparent until its thinned portion finishes covering the ciliary processes. Then it becomes pigmented a golden brown. The RPE stays true to itself (well-pigmented) over the whole path from posterior pole to the back of the iris.

The curved dotted line between the cornea and sclera marks the transition from the irregular fibers of the sclera to the more regular, clearer fibers of the cornea. Other anterior chamber angle details may be seen, including the modified vein (Schlemm canal) which drains aqueous humor from the eye.

The muscles of the ciliary body are shown in red: the muscle which is important for accommodation is the circular muscle. As shown in Figure 42, when the circular muscle contracts, tension on the lens capsule is released and the capsule tightens to deform the lens to increase its focal power for near vision.

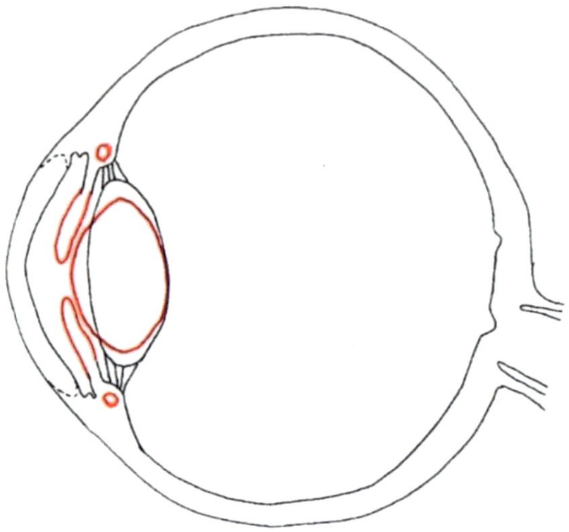

Figure 42  Accommodation:  in red, increased lens curvature shown, pupil constricted

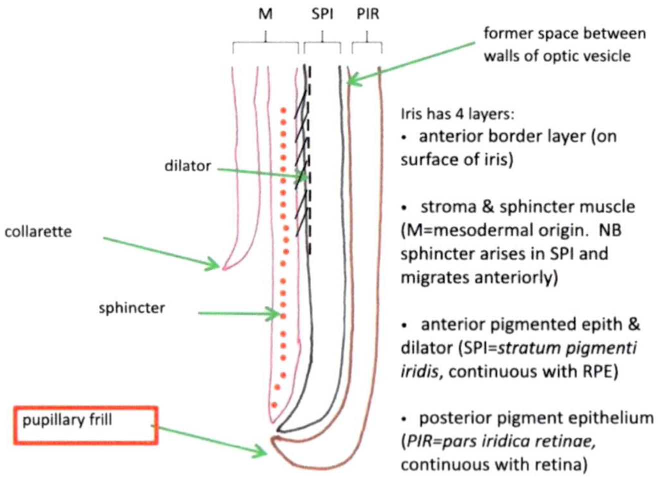


Figure 43  Four layers of iris

Figure 43 shows the iris structure at the pupil. Here the four layers of the iris are easily seen: on the left are the two layers contributed by the neural crest and mesoderm (see the bracket 'M' at the top). Behind them are the two layers contributed by the optic cup, with the part coming from the retinal pigment epithelium (RPE) marked by the bracket 'SPI' at the top, and the part coming from the retina itself marked by the bracket 'PIR'.

The muscles which operate the pupil are shown: the sphincter muscles make the pupil smaller, while the dilator muscles (surprise!) make the pupil larger. The frontmost layer of the iris usually stops short of the pupil margin, creating the collarette, which can be recognized easily. If there is any persistence of the pupillary membrane (take a look at Figure 40), the cobwebby material may be seen to anchor at the collarette (not captured in Figure 40). At the bottom of Figure 43, you can see how the golden brown pupillary frill is caused by the retinal part of the iris on its back surface doing sort of an end-run around the RPE portion. Figure 44 is a good photo of the pupillary frill.

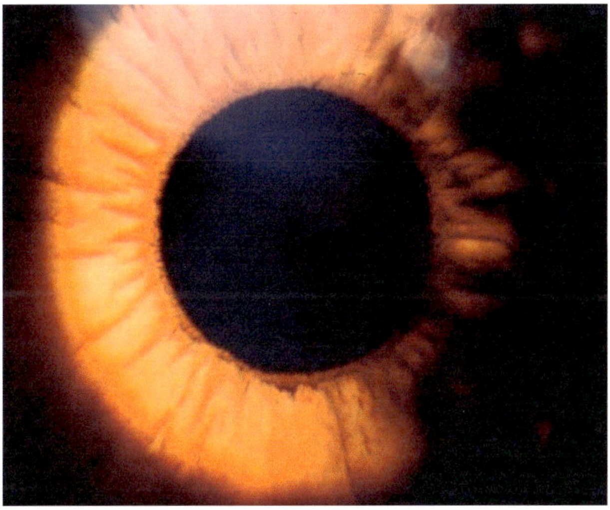

**Figure 44 Pupillary frill**

This golden pupillary frill is the most anterior part of the retina.

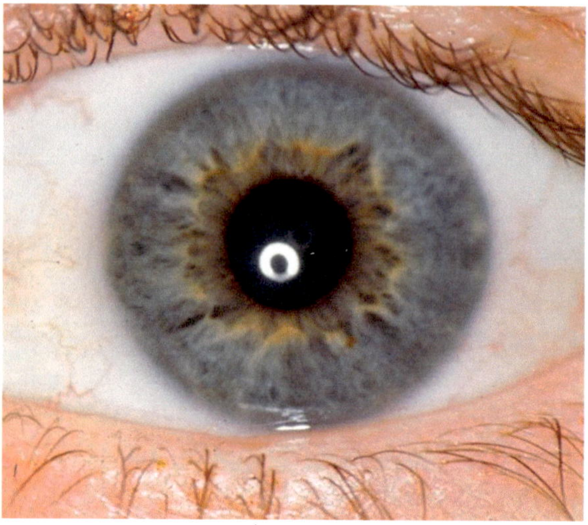

Figure 45 Visible collarette in blue iris

Here we can see the boundary between the front layer of the iris and the second layer of the iris: this boundary is called the collarette. This feature is present in most irises, but is easier to see in blue irises, because of the darker, deeper layer.

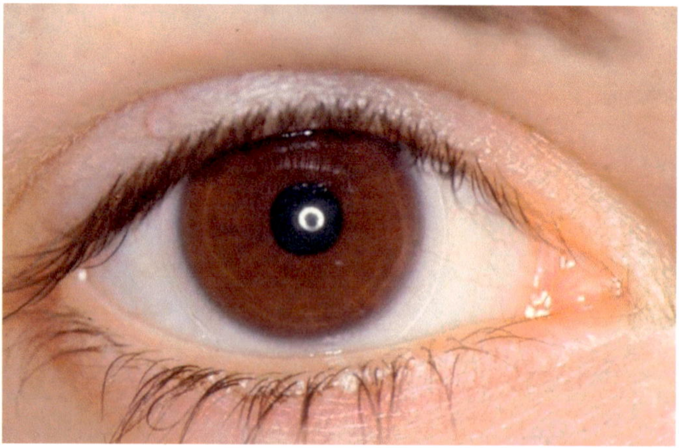

Figure 46 Brown iris with contraction furrows

With a brown iris, the melanocytes in the front two layers of the iris contain much melanin. By the way, this person is wearing a contact lens. For people with brown irises, sometimes contraction furrows may be seen as concentric rings on the iris surface toward the iris periphery. These are caused by dilation and constriction of the pupil, and are of no consequence.

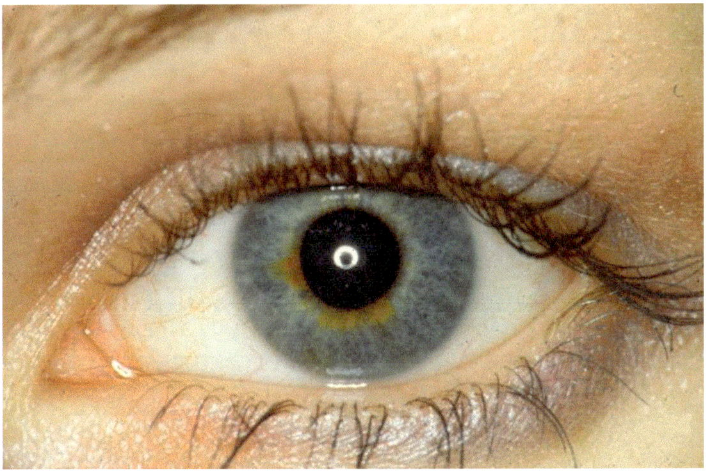

**Figure 47 Blue iris with deeper pigment visible**

This iris has relatively little melanin in the melanocytes of the frontmost of the two front layers. It is possible to see that the second deeper layer does have more melanin in its melanocytes, because you can observe the more pigmented layer close to the edge of the pupil.

## PIGMENT IN THE RODS AND CONES (THE PHOTORECEPTORS)

Photopigment is found in the outer segments of the rods and cones. Photopigment which has not been exposed to light, consists of a vitamin A compound called RETINAL and a protein (OPSIN). In rods, photopigment is in disc-shaped membranes which are separated from the cell membrane, while in cones, the photopigment is found in comb-shaped infoldings of the cell membrane. The cones of our retina possess three different opsins, and respond differently to light of different wavelengths. Red-sensitive cones have a peak sensitivity at 564 nanometers, green-sensitive cones at 534 nm, and blue-sensitive cones at 420 nm.

All rods have a peak sensitivity to light of wavelength 498 nm, a greenish-blue color. The rods are relatively insensitive to longer wavelengths, such as the red end of the spectrum, so night vision is less affected by red light. As vitamin A is a key component of photopigment, vision may be affected by vitamin A deficiency. Because rods are the most numerous photoreceptors, night vision is often the first to be affected by it.

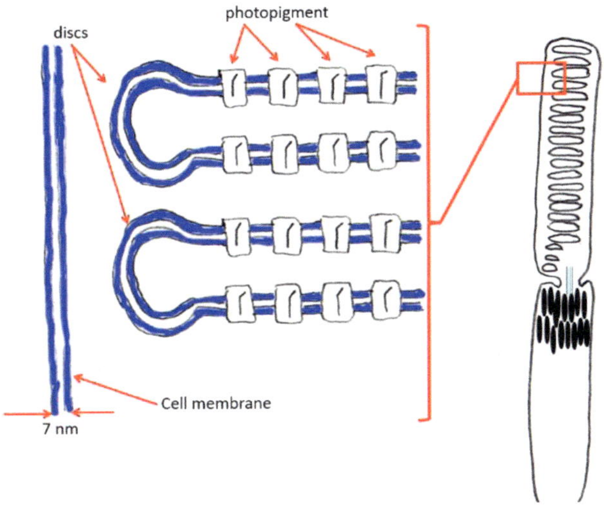


**Figure 48 Photopigment embedded in discs of rod photoreceptor**

The discs of rod photopigment (in the receptor outer segment) have the photopigment embedded in their membrane. The white blocks represent the protein opsin, and the bent black lines represent RETINAL, the light-sensitive vitamin A compound. When the photopigment captures a photon, the RETINAL changes its shape from the bent shape shown here to a straight shape, and is now called RETINOL. This change in shape causes the receptor to send signals to its axon, starting the visual process. The RETINOL detaches from the opsin and travels to the retinal pigment epithelial (RPE) cell where it is converted back to RETINAL, which is recycled via the inner segment to the receptor outer segment to rejoin with opsin. During periods of darkness, some aged discs, which are about 10 nanometers thick, are shed and digested by the RPE. The average RPE cell consumes about 4000 discs per day.

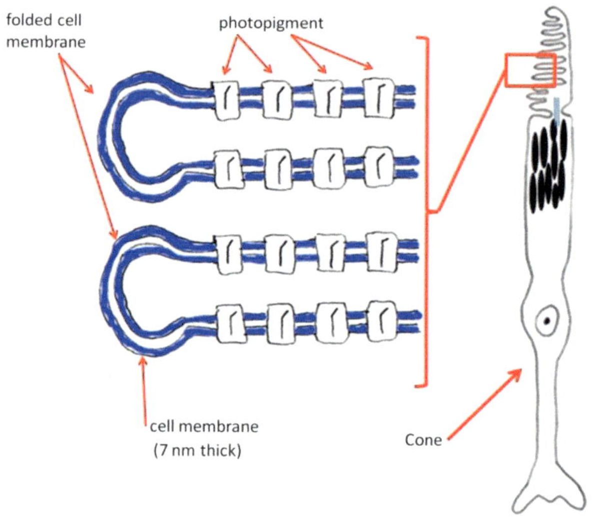


Figure 49  Photopigment embedded in membrane of cone

The story for cones is much the same, except that the photopigment is contained in a series of infoldings of the cell membrane (rather than the discs in rods).  New photopigment layers are generated in the inner segment of the photoreceptor, and migrate toward the outer segment.

# Chapter 3 CIRCULATION OF THE EYE

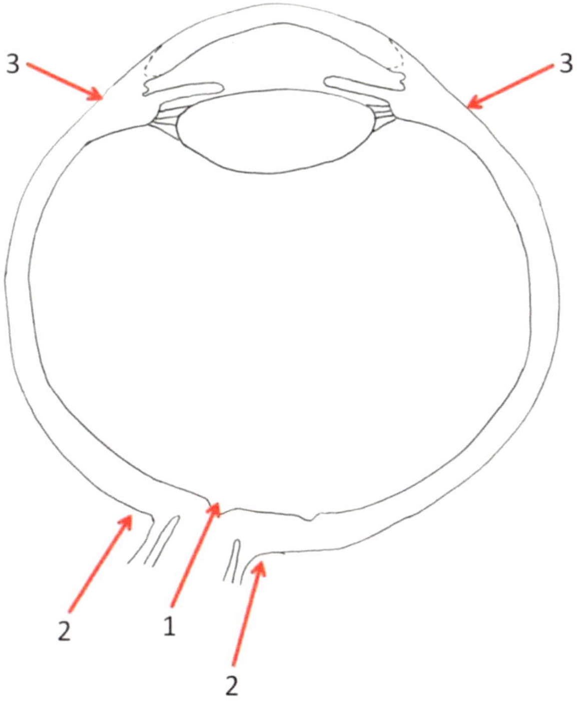


Figure 50 Vascular inputs to eye

Maintaining the retina takes a lot of energy, as it is a part of the brain. Most of it is sandwiched between two generous blood supplies: the CHOROIDAL circulation and the RETINAL circulation. Some compromises are necessary in the macular area, because blood vessels there can interfere with vision. An extensive blood supply is needed for the continuous production of aqueous, which fills the anterior chamber and drains out at the angle.

As seen in Figure 50, the retina receives blood from the central retinal circulation (1) and from the choroid, which receives a strong blood supply from vessels which enter in a ring around the nerve head, the short posterior ciliary arteries (2). The ciliary body has a strong blood supply (3) from blood vessels which go through the sclera by the ciliary body (the anterior ciliary arteries), and also from the long posterior ciliary arteries, which run forward between the choroid and sclera from the positions marked as 2. These branches are all from the ophthalmic artery, which is the first branch to leave the internal carotid artery after it enters the skull.

## RETINAL CIRCULATION

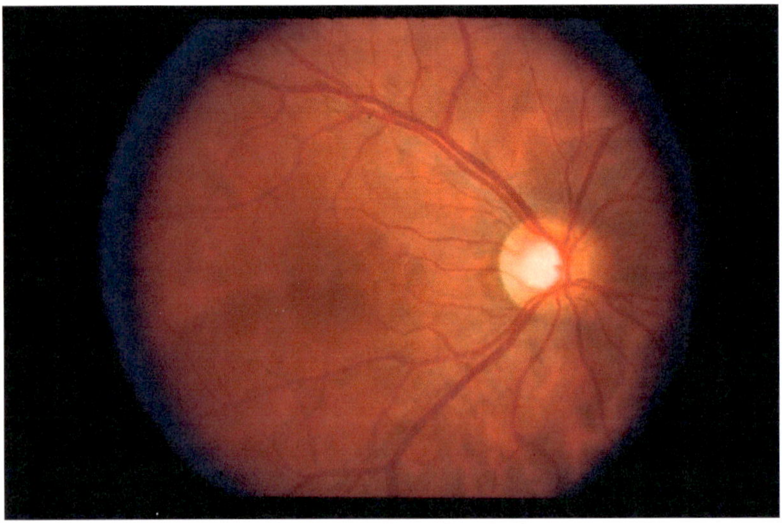

**Figure 51 Retinal circulation**

Here we see the retinal circulation in a right eye. The central retinal artery enters at the nerve head (on the right of the image) and sends branches over the retinal surface, avoiding the foveal area (slightly more pigmented region to the left of the nerve head). Some dimensions may be useful here:

- Nerve head diameter: 1500 micrometers (1.5 millimeters)
- Central retinal artery diameter: 150 micrometers (not visible here)
- Smallest vessels crossing disc margin: 15 micrometers

There are no retinal capillaries within a 250 micrometer radius of the foveal center. The retinal veins are darker and wider than the arteries.

The normal retina is transparent and the thickness of a sheet of paper. At the center of this nerve head, you may see a pattern of gray polygons (bundles of Ganglion Cell Axons) with white lines (the lamina cribrosa) between them. This pattern is visible in nerve heads which have a deep cupping. In diabetes, there may be aneurysms, hemorrhages, or growth of new blood vessels. In hypertension, constriction of arterioles may be seen; hardening of arterioles may make them compress underlying veins. If there is swelling of the retina for any reason, it will become opaque.

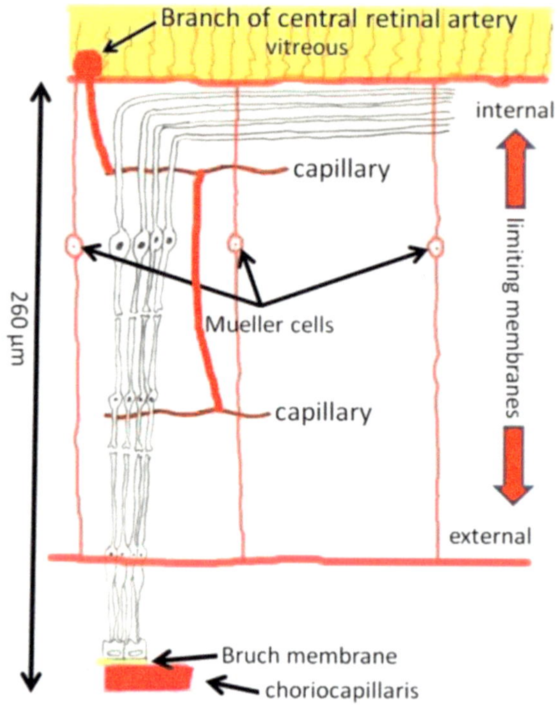


Figure 52 Capillary connections in retina

This is a view of the blood supply within the retina and away from the foveal center. The central retinal vessels supply capillaries inside the retina. Only two layers of capillaries are shown here; closer to the nerve head, there are two more capillary layers. At the bottom of Figure 52, receptor outer segments are seen inserted into retinal pigment epithelial cells, which themselves rest on Bruch membrane (yellow). Intraretinal capillaries are absent from the foveal center, so the retina there is dependent on the choroid for its blood supply. The rest of the retina is literally sandwiched between choroidal and retinal blood supply.

The Mueller cells produce both the internal and external limiting membranes of the retina, giving the neuroretina some structural framework. The Mueller cells also produce the strands of collagen which run through the vitreous and anchor it to the internal limiting membrane.

## CHOROIDAL CIRCULATION

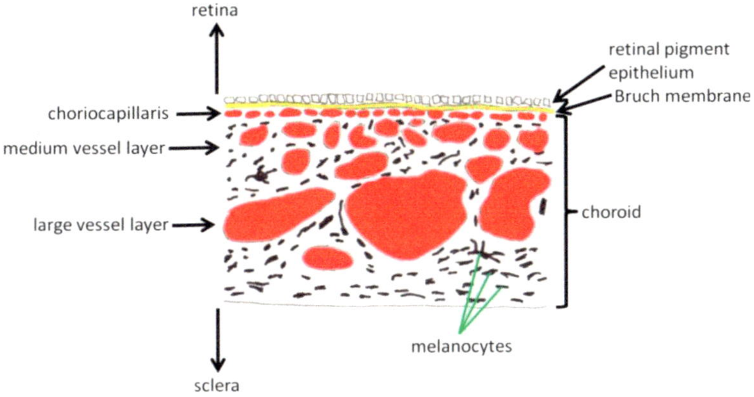


**Figure 53 Choroidal circulation**

This view shows how intensely vascular the middle layer (choroid) of the eye is. The choroid is 275 micrometers thick. Because the middle layer of the eye is thick and highly vascular and the sclera is not stretchy, expansion and contraction of the choroid with each heartbeat causes the intraocular pressure to go up and down, synchronous with the heartbeat. Many pigment cells (melanocytes) are found in the choroid, giving it a bluish color: hence it is referred to as the uveal tract (uva referring to a blue grape). Bruch membrane (yellow) separates the choriocapillaris from the retinal pigment epithelial layer. The vigorous blood flow through the choroid also helps dissipate heat from the images formed on the retina (consider the heat you feel on your hand when you image the sun on it with a magnifying glass). The image of the sun on the retina is about half a degree in size, which translates to 150 micrometers or 75 cones. This concentration of energy can damage the retina, which is why prolonged looking at the sun is dangerous, and sunglasses are recommended.

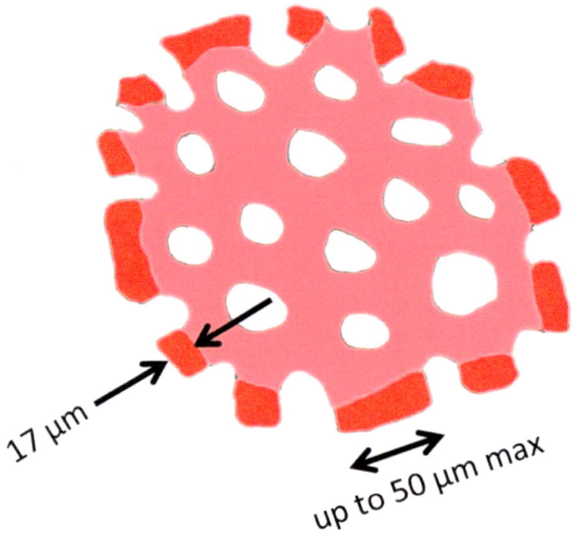


**Figure 54 Choriocapillaris detail**

Just below (and external to) the Bruch membrane is the choriocapillaris, the innermost part of the choroid.

Here is a schematic view of a small section of the choriocapillaris. It is a layer of merged capillaries which is about 17 micrometers thick. The width of the capillaries may be up to 50 micrometers (an average capillary is otherwise around 6 micrometers in diameter). The prime function of this layer is the nourishment of the photoreceptors and retinal pigment epithelium.

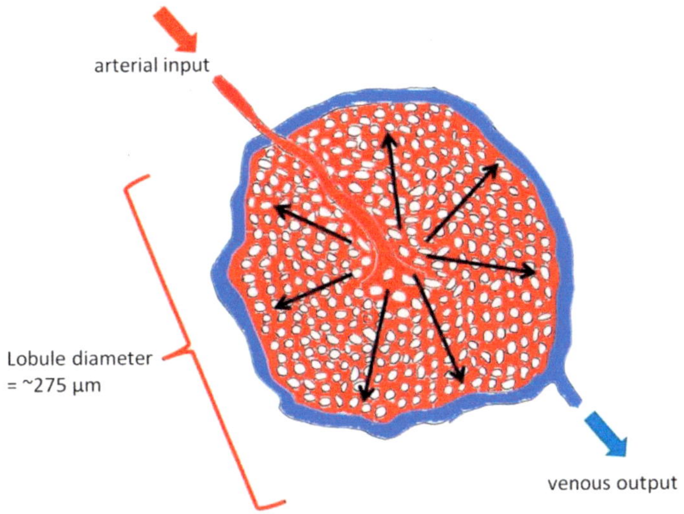


**Figure 55 Lobular circulation of choriocapillaris**

The choriocapillaris is arranged into functional units called lobules (like wagon wheels). Arterial blood is delivered to the center and travels outward, to be collected in the venous output at the edge.

# Chapter 4 THE VISUAL PATHWAY

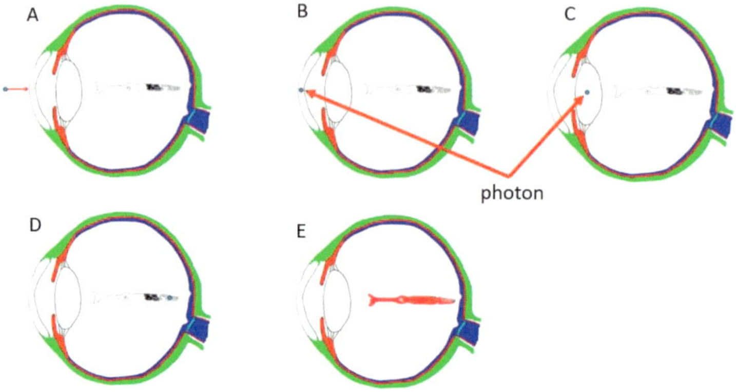


**Figure 56 Path of photon to photoreceptor**

Here is how vision begins:

A single photon is capable of starting the visual process!

A: The photon (a particle of light) is travelling toward the eye at $3 x 10^{10}$ centimeters per second (1080 x $10^6$ kilometers per hour or 675 x $10^6$ miles per hour.
B: As the photon enters the cornea, it slows down to 2.24 $x10^{10}$ centimeters per second
C: The photon passes through the lens
D: The photon passes through the neuroretina, to be captured by pigment in the photoreceptor outer segment. The photoreceptor and photopigment orientation increase the likelihood of capturing a photon
E: Once the photoreceptor captures a photon, its membrane has electrical and chemical changes

The electrical changes are passed on to the next cell in the visual pathway, the bipolar cell (Figure 57)

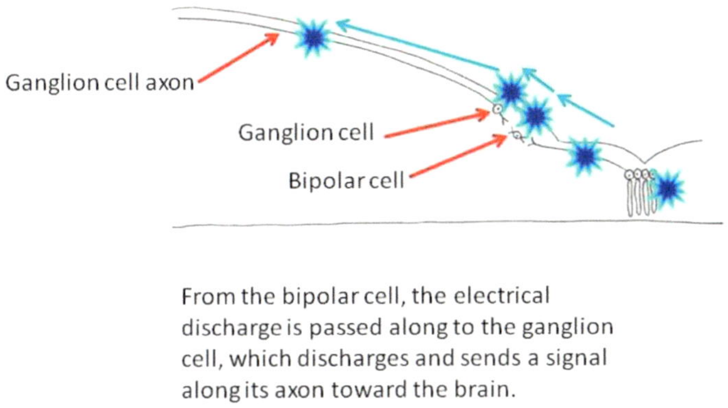


Figure 57 Path of nerve impulses to ganglion cell axon

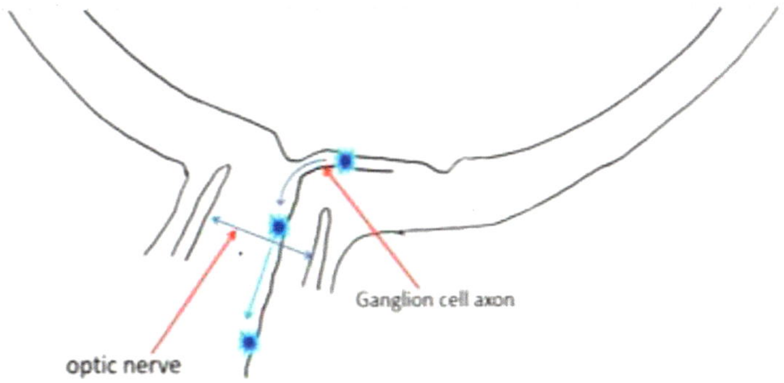


Ganglion cell axon joins up with over a million other axons to form the optic nerve, which is on its way to the midbrain.

Figure 58 Path of nerve impulses to optic nerve

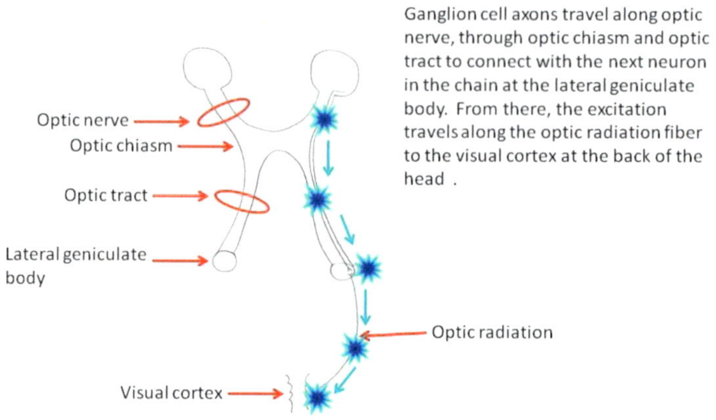


**Figure 59 Path of nerve impulses to visual cortex**

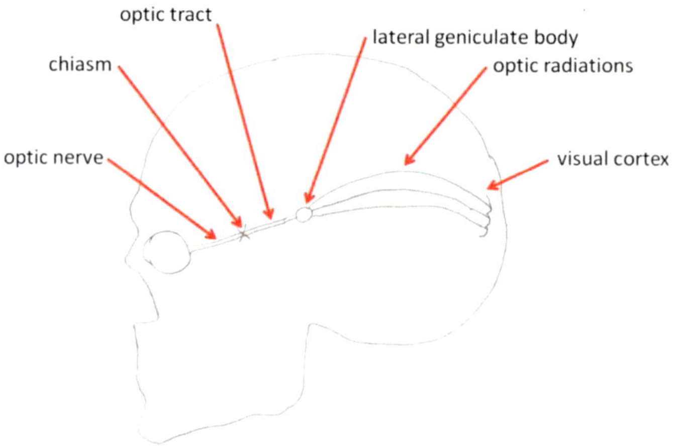


**Figure 60 Side view of visual pathway**

Here is the fully-developed visual pathway: it extends from the front of the head to the back. The embryonic brain tissue which became the retina sent nerve fibers (the ganglion cell axons) which found their way from the retina, travelling all the way through the rest of the developing brain from the eyeball to the lateral geniculate body. On their way, the ganglion cell axons travelled in the optic nerve, and through the chiasm (where some of them crossed over to the other side of the brain) and optic tract to reach the lateral geniculate body. From the lateral geniculate body, the optic radiation fibers carried the visual information to the visual cortex in the occipital lobe at the back of the head. (The back of the head is referred to as the occiput.) The map of the cells in the visual cortex parallels the map of their respective photoreceptors in the retina. The macula is represented by cortical cells at the very tip of the occiput, while cells farther away from the occiput represent more peripheral retina.

For some people with migraines, a wave of electrical stimulation begins at the posterior part of the visual cortex (where the fibers from the macula end), and moves forward toward parts of the visual cortex which serve the peripheral retina. This explains why, during a migraine attack, people see a pattern of flashing lights in the center of their visual field, and the pattern then expands toward the peripheral visual field.

The skull develops after the formation of the brain is nearly complete and the portion of central nervous system which becomes the retina is now housed in the orbit, and somewhat isolated from the rest of the brain, which is inside the skull. The orbit is the spherical hollow at the front of the skull, and the eye occupies about 30% of its volume: the rest of the orbit is filled with fat and muscles for eye movement.

## CLINICAL IMPLICATIONS

Because the visual pathway runs from the front of the head to the back, there is a strong possibility that events such as tumors or hemorrhages will impact vision in some way. Testing of visual functions such as pupil and eye movement, as well as visual field may give useful information on the location of problems along the visual pathway.

In hyperthyroidism, swelling of the muscles in the orbit may cause the eye to be pushed forward, which can cause problems with eye movements.

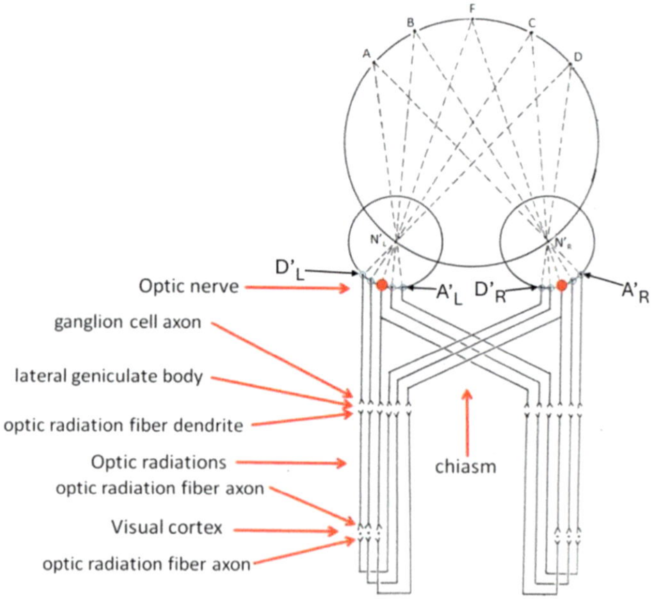


**Figure 61 Schematic of visual pathway**

Figure 61 is a schematic view of the visual pathway, viewed from the top. $N'_L$ and $N'_R$ represent the nodal points of the eyes: any light ray hitting the retina passes through the nodal points of that eye. The filled red circles at the back of each eye represent the foveas. Retina which lies toward the nose from the fovea is nasal retina, while retina which lies toward the temple (side of the head) is temporal retina. In humans, roughly half of the Ganglion Cell Axons (those from the nasal retina) cross to the other side of the brain. The other half, from the temporal retina, do not cross. This late development in the evolution of the visual system is what makes binocular vision possible in humans. This region of crossing and non-crossing axons is referred to as the Chiasm because it looks like an 'X'. The pituitary gland lies just below the chiasm. An enlarging pituitary tumor may compress some of the crossing axons and reduce their function. This may result in a visual field loss affecting the temporal visual field of each eye. The internal carotid arteries are just lateral to the chiasm. If they develop aneurysms, this may affect the non-crossing axons there. After passing through the chiasm, the ganglion cell axons end at the lateral geniculate body, where they connect to the beginning of the optic radiation fibers, which carry the visual impulses to the visual cortex at the back of the head.

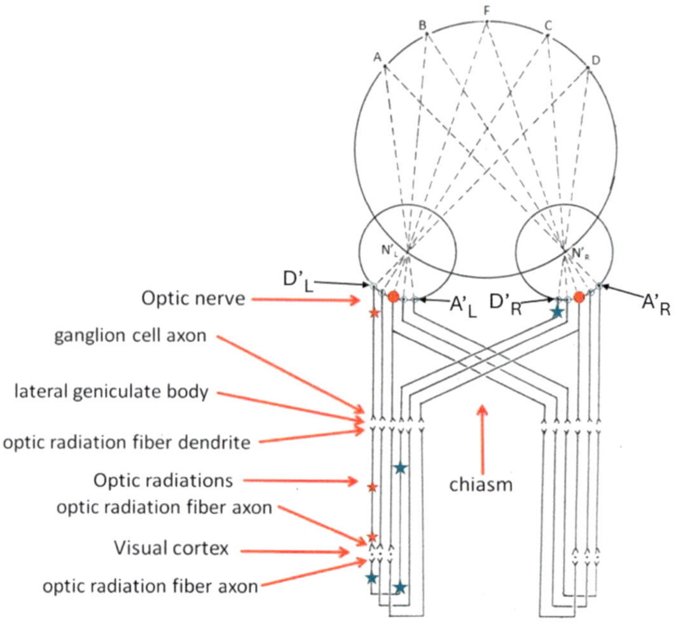


**Figure 62 Pathway for impulses to left visual cortex**

The person in Figure 62 is looking straight at the point F so the fovea of each eye is lined up with the image of F (filled red circles on retina). The point D (which is to the right of F) is imaged on the retinas as $D'_L$ and $D'_R$. Impulses generated by image $D'_L$ travel directly from the left eye to the left visual cortex, while those from image $D'_R$ in the right eye cross over at the chiasm on their way to the left visual cortex. Both sets of impulses end up at the same cell in the left visual cortex. $N'_L$ and $N'_R$ represent the nodal points of the eye.

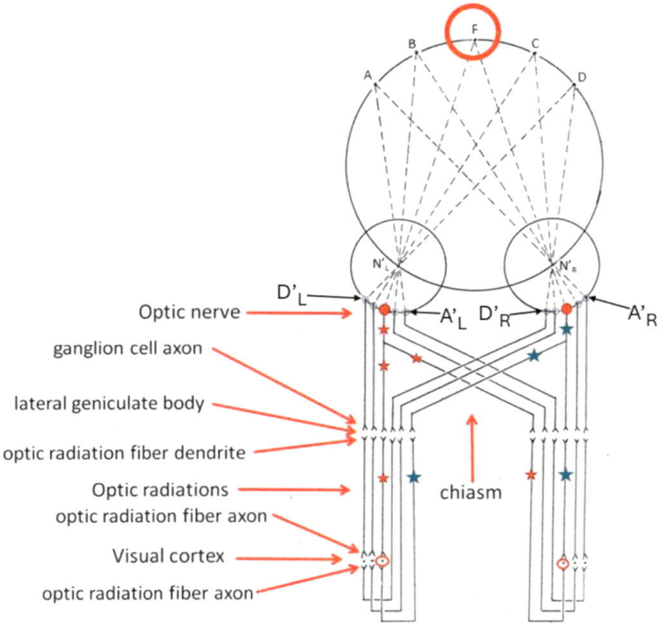


**Figure 63 Pathway of impulses from foveas**

When you look directly at the point 'F' as shown in Figure 63, you line up the fovea of each eye (filled red circles on the retinas) with the image of 'F'. While impulses from temporal retina (retina toward the temple from the fovea) DO NOT cross at the chiasm, and impulses from the nasal retina (retina toward the nose from the fovea) DO cross at the chiasm, the fovea itself is represented on BOTH SIDES of the visual cortex. This is a reason why your vision with both eyes open is sharper than with either eye alone.

Note that objects C and D are in the right visual field, and will wind up stimulating two brain cells in the left visual cortex. Objects A and B are in the left visual field, and wind up stimulating two brain cells in the right visual cortex. The object F stimulates brain cells in both the right and left visual cortex. This is why, though there are only five objects in the visual field, there are six stimulated brain cells: this is because the object F stimulates two brain cells, one on each side of the visual cortex. The retinal points stimulated by objects A, B, F, C, and D are termed CORRESPONDING POINTS. Each pair of corresponding points is associated with the same visual direction, and gives rise to perception of a single image.

As mentioned, the layout of brain cells in the visual cortex has a similar roadmap to that of the receptors in the retina. In humans, the nasal retinal cells and their Ganglion Cell Axons develop weeks before their temporal counterparts, reflecting their earlier position in the evolution of the visual system. It's all quite remarkable!

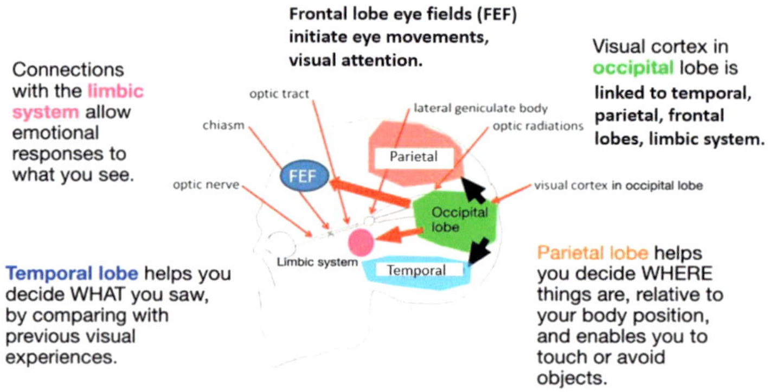


**Figure 64 Vision involves all lobes of the brain**

Although it takes only 6.3 milliseconds for impulses from the eye to reach the visual cortex, the subsequent processing of visual information involves all lobes of the brain. It takes about 180 milliseconds for you to realize that something has changed in your visual field. If you project images on a screen at 24 frames per second (standard in movie theaters), then the visual system is presented with a new image every 41 milliseconds. This is less than one fourth of the reaction time of the visual system. Your brain doesn't know that a new image has been presented, so it simply assumes that the image itself has moved.

# Chapter 5 TYPES OF ACUITY

## LETTER ACUITY (OR VISUAL ACUITY)

The letters for the visual acuity chart are constructed so that each element of the letter is the same size as the next. So, the standard 'E' is a square which is five blocks on each side. Other visual acuity charts may be made of circles with a gap equal to the gap shown on the right side of the 'E'. The circles are presented with the gap in different positions, and your task on circle charts is to see if you can tell where the gap is. Still other charts may use images of familiar objects, such as sailboats, hats, etc.

Standard Notation:

20/20: you see at 20 feet what the average observer sees at 20 feet. Each piece of the letter E is 1 minute of arc (1/60 degree) in size

20/40: you see at 20 feet what the average observer sees at 40 feet. Each piece of the letter E is 2 minutes of arc (2/60 degree) in size.

20/200: you see at 20 feet what the average observer sees at 200 feet. Each piece of the letter E
is 10 minutes of arc (10/60 degree) in size.

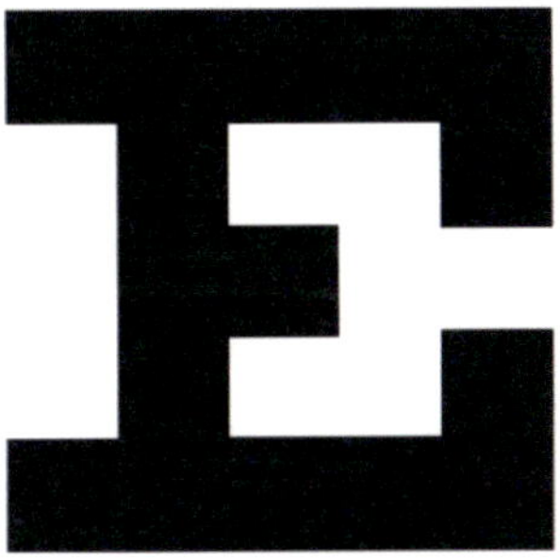

Figure 65 The Big E

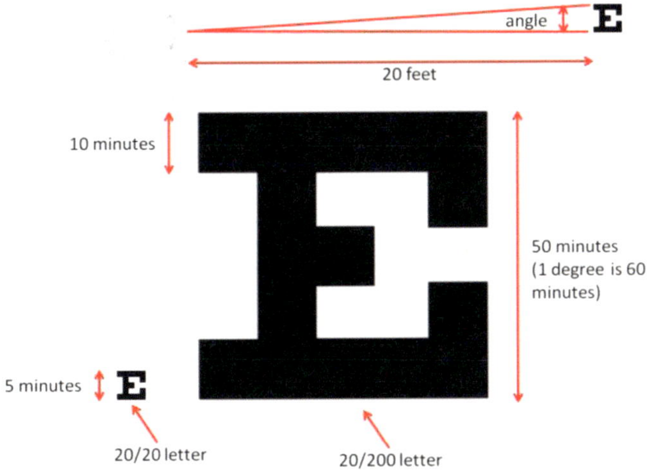


Figure 66 Visual angles for 20/20 and 20/200 E

Here is a comparison of the 20/20 'E' and the 20/200 'E' for viewing at 20 feet (6 meters). For the 20/20 'E', each part of the letter is 1 minute of arc in size. This means that, when the chart is shown at the correct distance (20 feet), each part of the letter makes an angle at the eye of 1 minute, or 1/60 of a degree. So, for the 20/20 letter, the total size of the angle will be 5 x 1 = 5 minutes. For the 20/200 letter, each part makes an angle of 10 minutes, so the whole letter will give an angle of 5 x 10 = 50 minutes, or almost a whole degree, since 1 degree = 60 minutes.

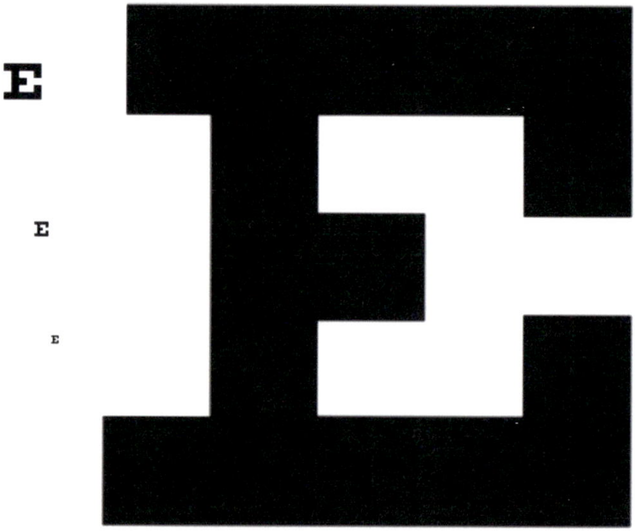

Figure 67 Visual angles for near and distance acuity measurement

The top left E, viewed from a distance of 16 inches (40 cm), corresponds to a near visual acuity of 20/200. The smaller E on the left corresponds to a near visual acuity of 20/100, while the smallest E on the left corresponds to a near visual acuity of 20/40. The very large E on the right, if viewed from a distance of 20 feet (6 meters), corresponds to a distance visual acuity of 20/200.

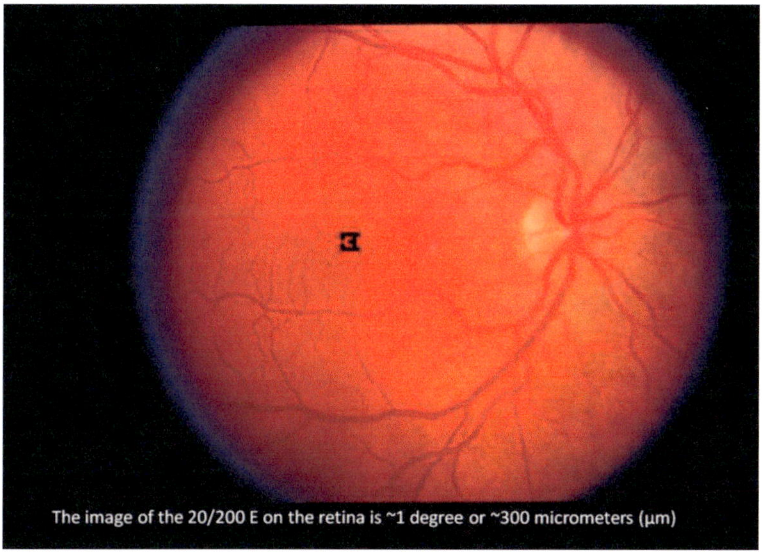


Figure 68 20/200 E imaged on the retina, to scale

The image of the 20/20 E is 1/10 the size of the 20/200 E. The 20/20 E image is only 25 micrometers across, the size of 4 red blood cells side by side. The largest letter on the visual acuity chart is slightly less than 1 degree in size, so all of the letters on the chart will be smaller than this: only one degree of visual field is necessary to read the whole chart.

You should NEVER assume your eye and visual system are healthy just because you can read all the letters on the acuity chart! Many diseases can affect the visual field; for example, glaucoma, brain tumours, and retinal infections and still leave the central one degree of field intact. The whole visual system seems to be geared to hold onto that central one degree.

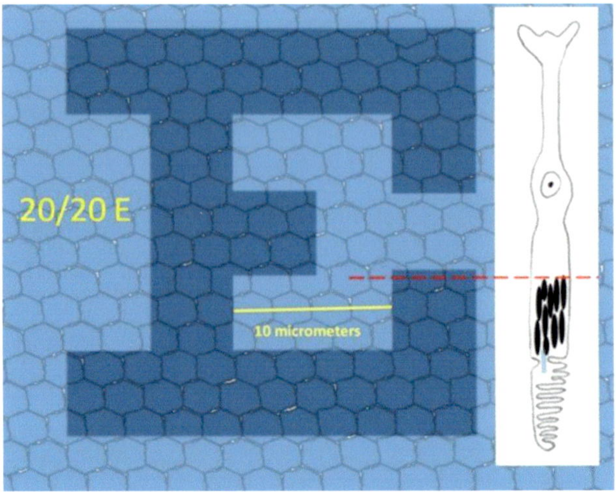


Figure 69 Size of 20/20 E on mosaic of foveal cones

Curcio (Journal of Comparative Neurology 1990;292:497) and her team obtained images of the retina at the level of the cones shown by the dashed red line on the right. The hexagons shown here are the size of the cone cross-sections. On average, there are about 4 cones per 10 micrometers. This allows a representation of a 20/20 E in relation to the photoreceptor pattern of the retina.

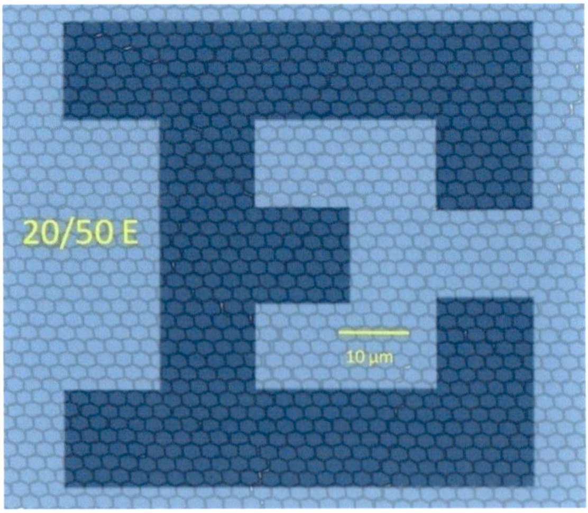


Figure 70 20/50 E on cone mosaic

Figure 70 is a representation of the retinal image of a 20/50 E against the pattern of foveal cones. (see Figure 69 for details).

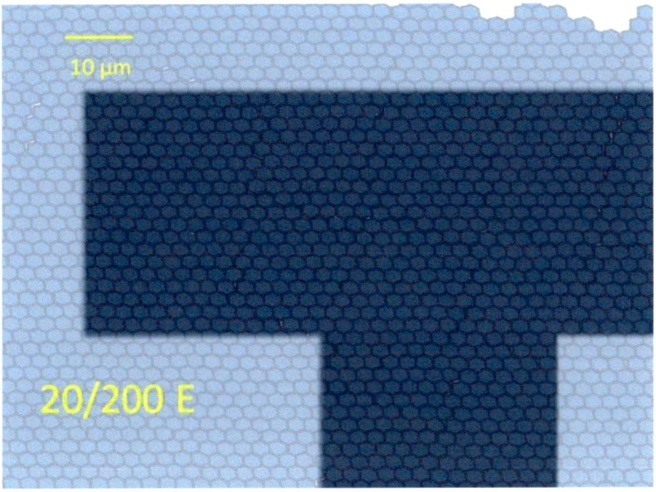


Figure 71 20/200 E on cone mosaic

A representation of a portion of the 20/200 E on the matrix of retinal cones. You can see that each part of the 20/200 E is falling on something like 20 cones. What this means in practical terms is that you can lose a fair number of cones (in macular degeneration, for example) and still have enough to be able to make out the letter. This is an example of the tremendous redundancy in the central nervous system!

The legal definition of blindness looks at two aspects of vision. EITHER a person has a visual acuity of less than 20/200 in their better eye OR a visual field width in the better eye of less than 20 degrees.

The minimum visual standards for driving in many jurisdictions are a visual acuity of 20/40 AND a horizontal field width of 120 degrees.

## Hooke and the minimum angle of resolution

In 1674, Hooke proposed that two stars had to be separated by an angle greater than 30 seconds (half a minute) for you to see them as two. One degree is 60 minutes, so half a minute is 1/120 of a degree. It was suggested that the images of these stars would have to land on the retina such that one image landed on one receptor, and the second would have to land on another receptor, with one unstimulated receptor between them.

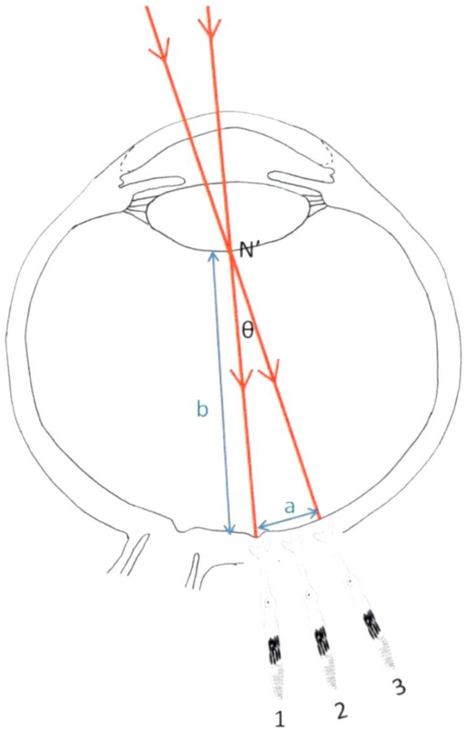


Figure 72 Hooke's idea on minimum angle of resolution

Let's say that theta (θ) is the angle between two stars which can just be resolved, that is, seen as two. Following Hooke's thinking, there should be one non-stimulated cone

(cone 2) between the two stimulated cones (cones 1 and 3). According to Curcio, the separation of 1 and 3 will be 5 micrometers. The distance from N' to the retina is 16 millimeters (16,000 micrometers). We can calculate the angle theta to have a tangent of 5/16,000. It works out to an angle of just a little over 1 minute, which is routinely used as the minimum angle of resolution in designing letters for visual acuity charts. By the way, the two nodal points of the eye (N and N') coincide, so only N' is shown.

## VERNIER ACUITY

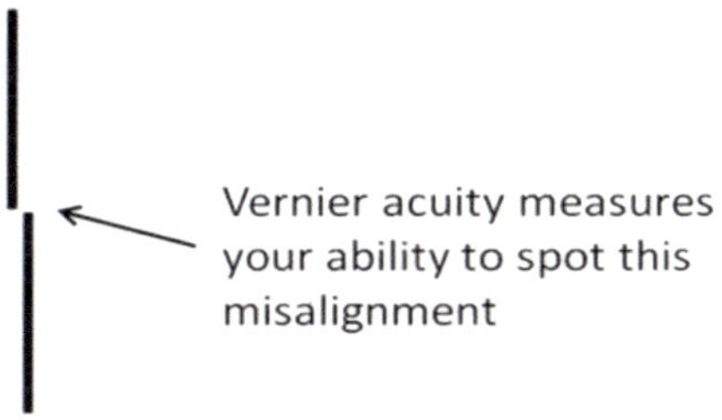


**Figure 73 Vernier acuity**

Vernier acuity is the ability to tell that two lines are not aligned with each other. It turns out that your best resolution for vernier acuity is more like 10 seconds of arc (1/6 of a minute, or 1/360 of a degree). In photographic terms, this resolution is better than the 'pixel count' of the retina. So, it turns out that there is a lot of neural processing of information higher in the brain than the retina.

## STEREO ACUITY

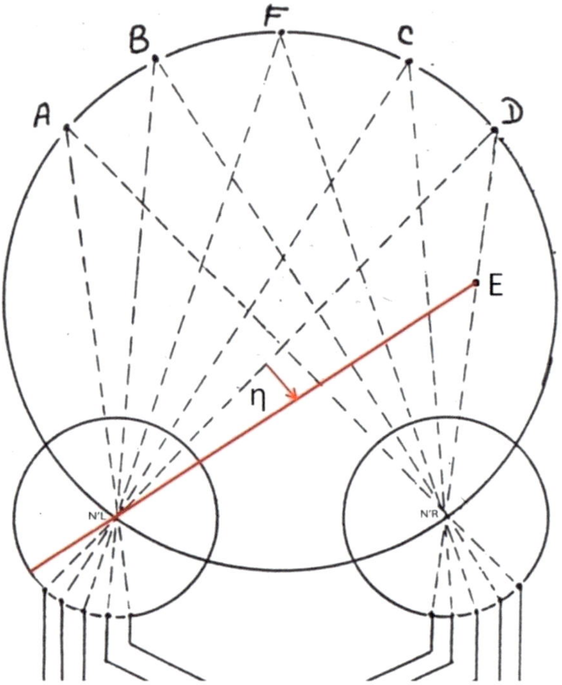


Figure 74 Stereo acuity

We've talked about letter acuity and vernier acuity. Now let's talk about stereo acuity. A point, E, has been added. The right eye will see it in the same direction as the point D, but the left eye will see it in a different direction. The angle marked by the Greek letter eta (η) is the difference between the direction in which E is seen by the left eye compared to the right. If E were moved back to D, then there would be no difference in the direction the left eye and the right eye saw it. The ability to recognize, using two eyes, that objects are at different distances from the observer is called stereopsis. A good observer could tell that E was closer than D when the angle eta (η) is as low as 5 seconds of arc and some observers can do even better.

This 5 second stereo acuity is much better (by a factor of 12) resolving power than the 1 minute of arc used for measuring visual acuity. N'L and N'R represent the nodal points of the eyes. The brain uses the slight differences in angle (such as eta) to develop a three-dimensional impression of the world, instead of seeing things doubled.

**Figure 75 Demonstration of stereopsis**

Here's a demonstration of stereopsis and the brain's ability to combine images neatly. Hold your finger between the book and your nose, and look at the tip of your finger. You will see a third set of circles above the tip of your finger. You will have the impression of looking down into a well, with the innermost circle being the farthest away of all three. Notice also that the circles appear to be spaced equally sidewise from each other. Your brain has interpreted the small differences between the two images, and built up a single three-dimensional image.

# Chapter 6 REFRACTION

This happens because light travels at different speeds in different substances. In water, light travels at 75% of its speed in air. This slowdown causes light rays to bend in a predictable way, and this is the basis for (among other things) the lenses which may be used to help people to see more clearly, and prisms which compensate for problems with binocular vision.

Did you know that the fossil record indicates that humans are related to fish which managed to 'walk' out of the ocean long ago? Since that event, the human eye has adapted considerably to life in air. If the human eye is immersed again in water, it loses 75% of its focal power, and underwater vision is seriously blurry. This problem is easily remedied by putting a thin layer of air in front of the eye (swim goggles or masks), which restore vision to normal.

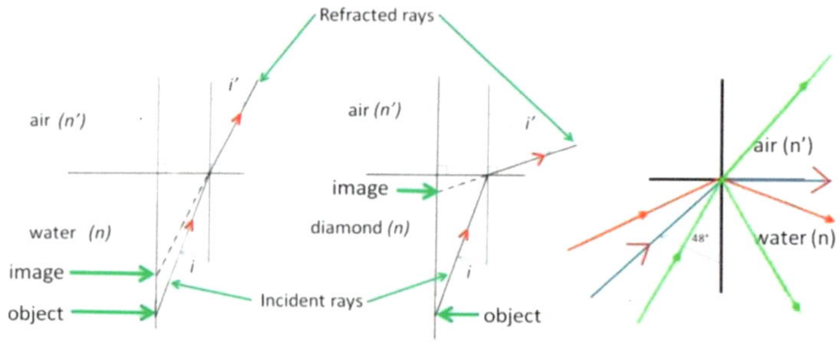


Figure 76 Rays travel from dense to rare medium; critical angle

The bending of light rays as they travel from one medium to another is called refraction. The speed of light in air is 3 x $10^{10}$ centimetres per second. Light travels more slowly in a medium denser than air. The ratio of the velocity of light in air to the velocity of light in a second medium is called the REFRACTIVE INDEX (n) of the medium. So, the refractive index of air is 1.0. The refractive index of water is 1.33. The refractive index of diamond is 2.4. Although the speed of light changes in a denser medium, the frequency of its component wavelengths is unchanged.

The diagrams above describe why objects under water (or diamond) appear to be closer to the surface than they really are. Light rays travelling from the object are bent as they enter air. Because of the bending of the rays, what you see (the image, shown by the dotted lines) lies closer to the surface. The vertical lines (normals) are at right angles to the surface: rays travelling from dense (water or diamond) to rare (air) will bend away from the normal.
Note that the rays travelling from diamond to air bend much further from the normal than those travelling from water to air. The greater the refractive index change from one material to another, the more bending of light rays happens.

In 1621, the Dutch astronomer and mathematician, Willebrord Snell studied the change in direction of light rays after they pass from one medium (such as water) into a second one (such as air). Snell found that the change in direction depended on the change in refractive index (n) from one medium to the other (n'). In the formula below, the letter i indicates the angle the incident ray makes with the normal to the surface, while the letter i' indicates the angle the refracted ray makes with the normal. Time for some more trigonometry, folks. The relationship between these angles and the refractive indices is shown in the formula

$$n \times \text{sine } i = n' \times \text{sine } i'$$

or if you prefer:

$$\frac{\text{sine } i}{\text{sine } i'} = \frac{n'}{n}$$

If you check the diagram against the formula, you will see that the water-to-air diagram, with its angle of incidence (i) = 20 degrees, correctly shows the angle of refraction (i') to be 27 degrees. For the diamond-to-air diagram, with the same angle of incidence of 20 degrees, the actual angle of refraction should be 55 degrees: the angle of refraction (shown as 70 degrees) has been exaggerated.

Looking at the diagrams above, you can see that if the angle of incidence (i) is increased enough, the refracted ray will wind up travelling PARALLEL to the interface between water/air or diamond/air. The angle of refraction (i') will be 90 degrees. This is shown by the blue ray in Figure 76. This angle of incidence is referred to as the critical angle, and works out to just over 48 degrees for a water/air interface. Any light rays hitting the interface with a greater angle of incidence will be REFLECTED at the interface (the red ray in Figure 76). This critical angle is why a submerged diver looking upward will see a circular window through which sunlight passes. The window is surrounded by reflections of objects below the surface.

The green ray shown in Figure 76 strikes the interface at an angle of 30 degrees: one part of the ray is refracted to an angle of 41 degrees, while a portion is reflected at an angle of 30 degrees. The proportion of light reflected at an interface depends on the difference between the refractive indices. For example, if you put a piece of glass with a refractive index of 1.523 under water with a refractive index of 1.33, there is little reflection from the glass, making it hard to see when it is under water.

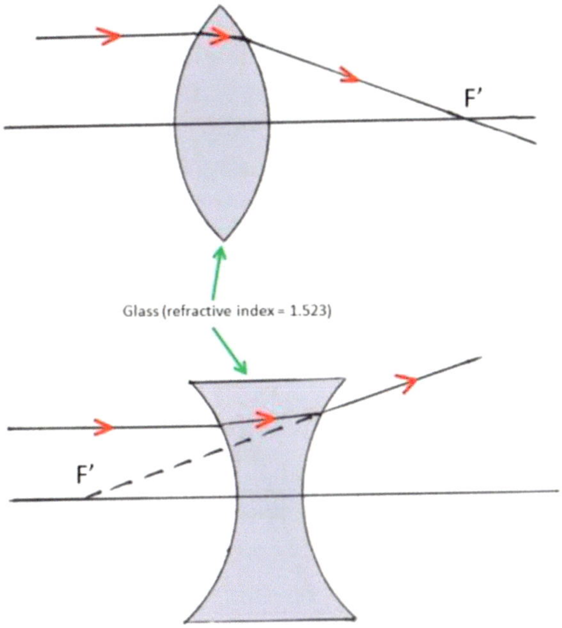


**Figure 77 How lenses work**

Light rays are bent (refracted) as they pass into and out of dense material such as glass. By arranging the curvature of the surfaces the rays pass through, the rays may be brought to a focal point (F'). In the case of a positive lens (shown at top of Figure 77), the image of a distant object is real, and can be shown on a screen. In the case of a negative lens (lower part of Figure 77), the image of a distant object is virtual. Although it cannot be shown on a screen, it can be seen by an eye on the right side of the lens! Light in nature is always diverging from its origin. The only way light can be made to converge is with the use of a positive lens or a concave mirror, so converging light is not encountered in nature. Rays of light coming from a great distance (such as a star) may be regarded as travelling parallel to each other (rays are really streams of photons).

In terms of the lenses that you may wear to clear up your distance vision, if you can see clearly at a distance of 20 feet or six meters, you will also be able to see infinitely-distant objects clearly. Light coming from a test target 20 feet away is actually diverging slightly, so an emmetropic person and would need a lens power of +0.16 diopters to clear up vision. This power is less than the accuracy of measurement, as the steps of power used in routine eye examinations are 0.25 diopters.

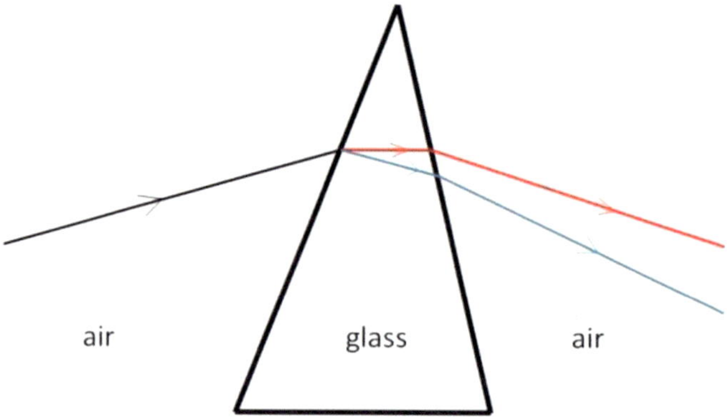


**Figure 78 How prisms work**

While lenses can change the way light focuses (either converging or diverging the rays), prisms can change the DIRECTION of light. An observer on the right side of this diagram would see objects as shifted upward.

White light is composed of all the colours of the rainbow. Each component of the ray of white light encounters a different velocity change as it enters and exits the prism, with the result that the white light is dispersed as shown: the red light is slowed less than the blue light, and the intervening colors (orange, yellow, green for example) will appear between the red and blue, forming a spectrum.

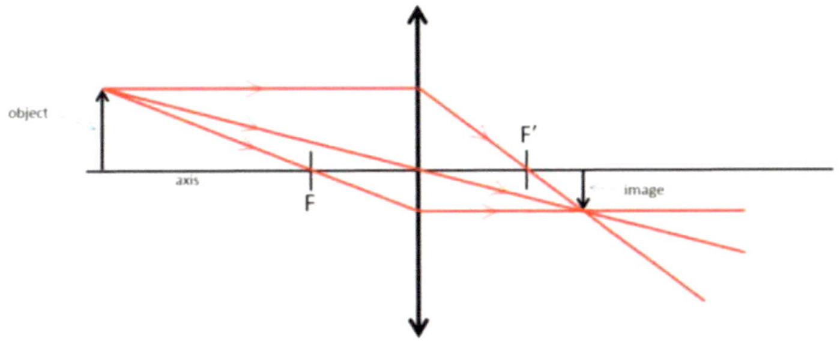


Figure 79 Thin lens forms real image

Here's a thin plus lens forming an image. A ray from the object which travels parallel to the axis will pass through the second focal point (F'), and a ray passing through the lens where the axis hits the lens will travel through without changing direction. A ray from the object which passes through the first focal point (F) will leave the lens running parallel to the axis. Where these three rays cross is the location of the image.

The eye's optical system is a positive one: all images on the retina will be upside down and reversed, so how do we see things right side up and not reversed? The retina is wired to solve the problem. Consider a right eye looking straight ahead: if light comes from a place to the right, it will fall on nasal retina and you will perceive the light as coming from your temporal visual field. The same goes for light directed upward into your eye: you will perceive it as coming from your inferior visual field: so really, the visual system turns your visual world the right way around.

## WHY OUR VISUAL WORLD ISN'T SEEN UPSIDE DOWN AND REVERSED.

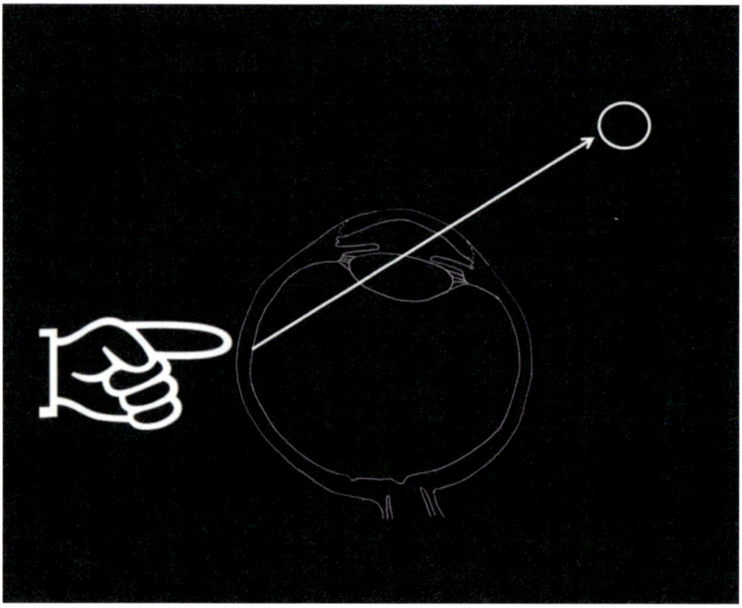

**Figure 80 How to produce a pressure phosphene**

Here's a little experiment to go with the story for Figure 79. Close both eyes and turn your eyes to the right. Now, with your finger apply gentle pressure through the eyelid at the outer corner of the eyelid of the left eye. You will see a ghostly bright partial circle of light toward your right. If you move your finger up and down on the eyelid, you will see that circle of light moving down and up on your right. Pressure from your finger is causing mechanical stimulation of the temporal retina. The result of this is that you will be aware of light to your right, as this is the place where light must originate in order to stimulate the area of temporal retina which you stimulated with your finger. What you are experiencing is called a pressure phosphene.

Seeing flashing lights when there is no light hitting the eye (photopsia) can have many causes, some innocent, some truly worrisome.

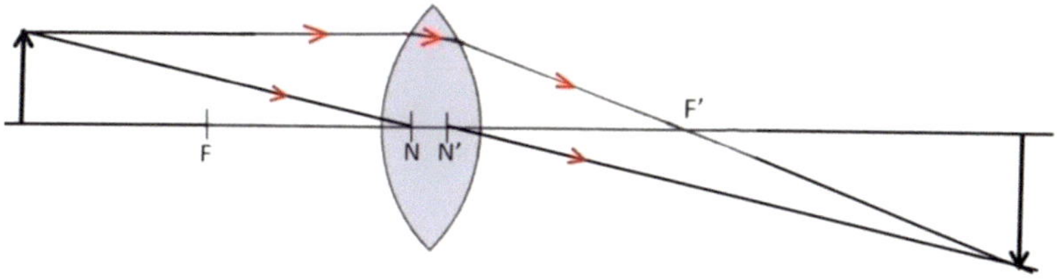


**Figure 81 Thick lens forms real image**

Here's the story for a thick lens, which could also represent the whole optical system of the eye. Optical systems possess two nodal points (N and N'). The property of nodal points is that a ray which is directed toward N will exit the optical system as though from N', with its direction unchanged. For the thin lens shown in Figure 79, the points N and N' coincide at the point where the axis passes through the thin lens. For the human eye, the nodal points coincide at the back surface of the crystalline lens. This nodal point business becomes interesting when we look at the orientation of photoreceptors in the retina. To increase the chance of catching a photon, the photoreceptors are all 'looking' at N'.

# OPHTHALMOSCOPE PRINCIPLE

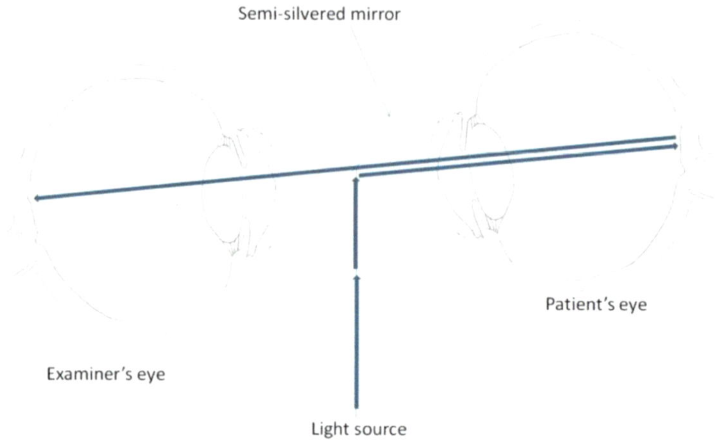


**Figure 82 Direct ophthalmoscope principle**

The 'red eye' appearance which shows up in photographs occurs because the camera flash and the camera lens are in line with each other. Instruments such as a direct ophthalmoscope use a similar system, including a light source and a semi-silvered mirror (a mirror which reflects, say, 50% of the light which hits it, and lets the rest go through). Using the mirror, the light is directed into the patient's eye. The mirror will also transmit light reflected from the back of the patient's eye into the eye of the examiner. Lenses may be placed between the two eyes to allow the examiner to focus on objects closer than the patient's retina. The direct ophthalmoscope gives a magnification of 15X, and a field of view of about 5 degrees (about the size of the optic nerve head).

If you wear glasses, you can get a look at the retina of your dog or cat without an ophthalmoscope.

- Place a light source somewhere behind your pet's head and aimed toward you.
- Move your own head around so the light reflects from your glasses into your pet's eye.

Dogs and cats are particularly interesting to look at this way, because they have a tapetum, a layer of crystals under the retina which strongly reflects light back out of the eye. The reason why animals with a tapetum have good night vision is because the reflection of light gives their photoreceptors twice the opportunity to catch photons.

## INDIRECT OPHTHALMOSCOPY

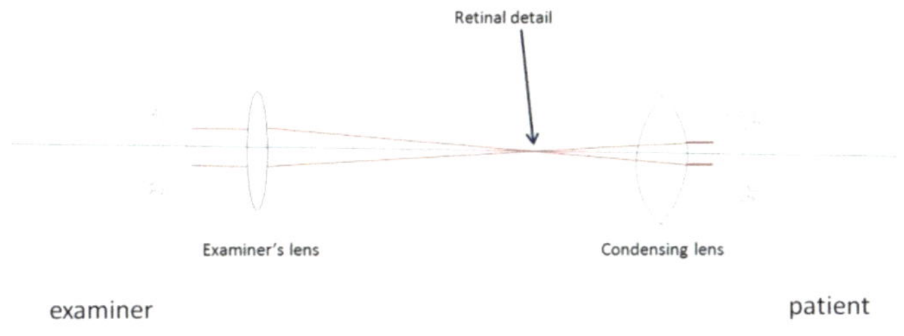


**Figure 83 Indirect opththalmoscope principle**

Indirect ophthalmoscopy gives a wider field of view. The examiner's light source is mounted on the head; a high-powered condensing lens (from +20 to +90 diopters) is held in front of the patient's eye; and the examiner looks through a lower-powered lens (around +2 diopters). For telescopes, rays entering and leaving the system are parallel to each other. Telescopes ordinarily have the higher-powered lens close to the user's eye, and the lower-powered lens at the

other end.
The indirect ophthalmoscope is like looking through the wrong end of a telescope: magnification is reduced (about 1/3 of that for the direct ophthalmoscope) and field of view is enlarged to about 30 degrees. Retinal detail is imaged at the point shown: this point is seen through the examiner's lens. If rays leaving the patient's eye are parallel to each other, he would have to be emmetropic, and for the examiner to see the retinal detail in focus when the parallel rays enter her eye, she would have to be emmetropic too! Small adjustments of lens position will clear up any blur.

## IMAGE FORMATION BY A PLUS LENS

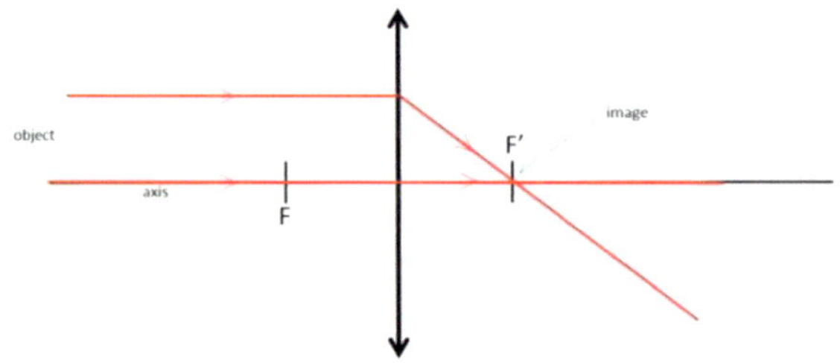


**Figure 84 Thin plus lens forms real image of distant object**

The following sequence of images shows all of the possible ways a plus lens may image a real object. This first image shows what happens when the real, physical object is as far away as possible to the left of the picture. The image will be found at the focal point of the lens, F'.

For example, if you have a hand magnifier, and you want to know its focal power, just take it outdoors in the sun and measure the distance from the lens to the in-focus image of the sun: focal power = 1/distance in meters. If your lens gives you an image of the sun at a distance of 10 centimeters from the lens, its focal power is 1/.1 = +10 diopters.

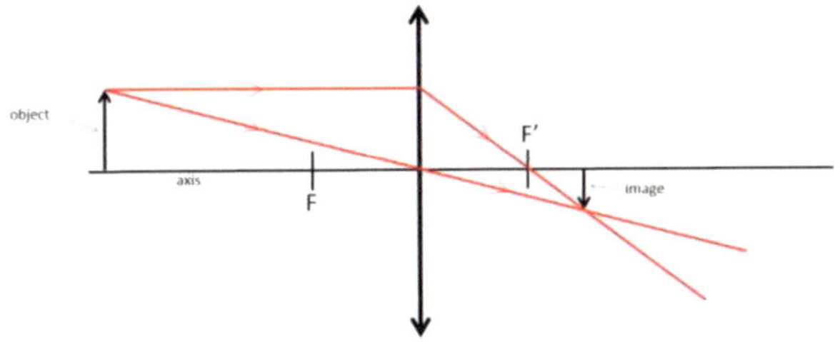


Figure 85 Thin plus lens gives larger image of nearby object

The real, physical object has been moved closer to the lens, and the image starts to get larger and moves from F' toward the right.

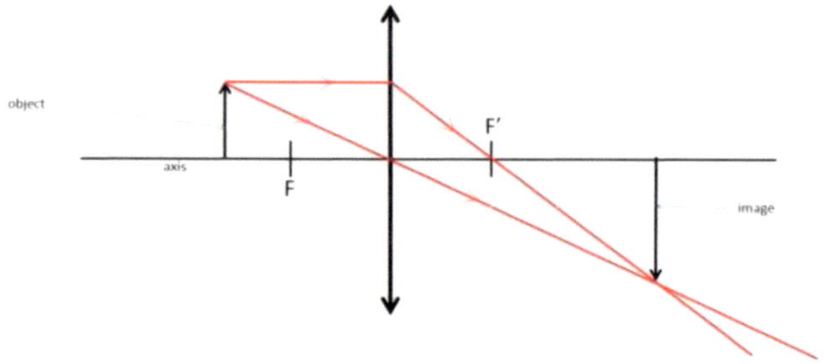


**Figure 86 Thin plus lens gives larger image of nearby object outside F**

Because the real object has been moved closer to F, the image gets larger still, and moves farther away toward the right side of the picture.

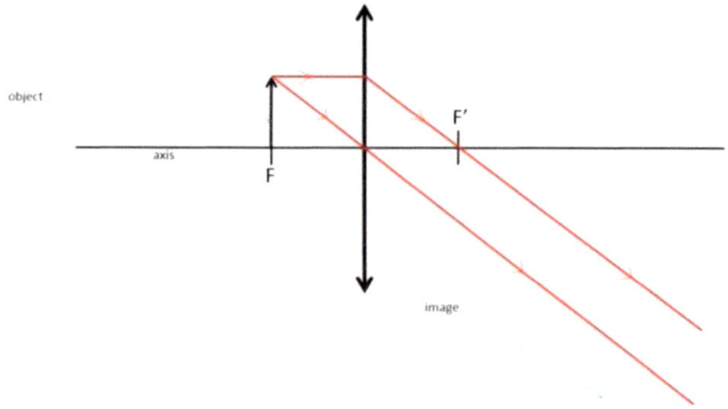


**Figure 87 Thin plus lens produces image at infinity for object at F of lens**

When the object is placed at F, the image will be found where the two rays intersect, that is, at a great distance to the right, because the emerging rays are parallel to each other. In optical terms, the image could be said to be at infinity, over to the right. An eye placed to the right of the lens would see the image as being over to the left. Because the emerging rays are parallel to each other, what the observer sees appears to be at a distance to the left of the diagram. While the real object was farther away from the lens than F, all of the images are real--that is, they could be shown on a screen. The image in this example COULD be shown on a screen, provided you could move it a great distance to the right...

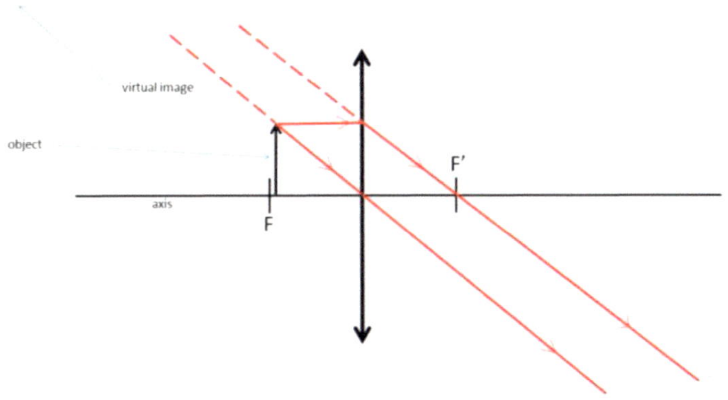


Figure 88 Thin plus lens produces virtual image of nearer object

Once the real object is brought closer to the lens than F, the rays leaving the lens are diverging, and are not actually going to intersect anywhere. The image has now become virtual. It cannot be shown on a screen. The location of the virtual image can be determined by tracing the rays backward to see where they intersect. In this case, the virtual image is going to be at a great distance to the left of the screen.

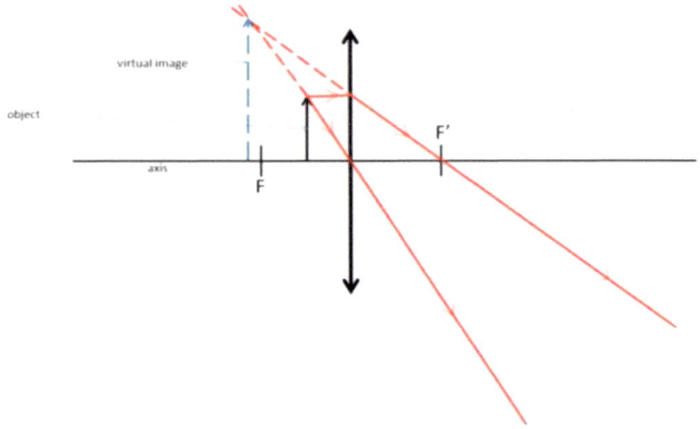


**Figure 89 Thin plus lens gives magnified virtual image of nearby object**

As the object moves closer still to the lens, the virtual image becomes smaller than that in Figure 88, and starts to approach the lens. Here's another experiment: if you are on the right-hand side of the lens, and bring the object just inside the position F, you will see the image magnified. This is the basis for hand-magnifiers like those used by Sherlock Holmes or your grandparent. A common lens power for a hand-magnifier is +8 diopters. The focal length for a +8 diopter lens is 1/8 meter = 12.5 centimeters (about 5 inches). If you hold the hand-magnifier closer than 5 inches from the object you are looking at, it will appear twice as large as the original.

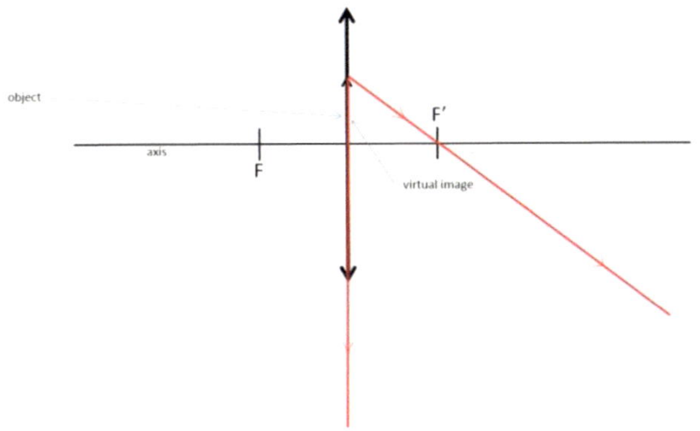


Figure 90 Thin plus lens gives image which coincides with the object

To complete the sequence, here is what happens when the object is RIGHT AT the lens. The virtual image, which has been approaching from a great distance to the left, and decreasing from a great size to nearly the same size as the object, now coincides with the object at the lens.

After going through this exercise, it appears that infinity over to the right of the diagram connects with infinity over to the left of the diagram; in other words, there is a continuity of the two infinities...or is it all the same?

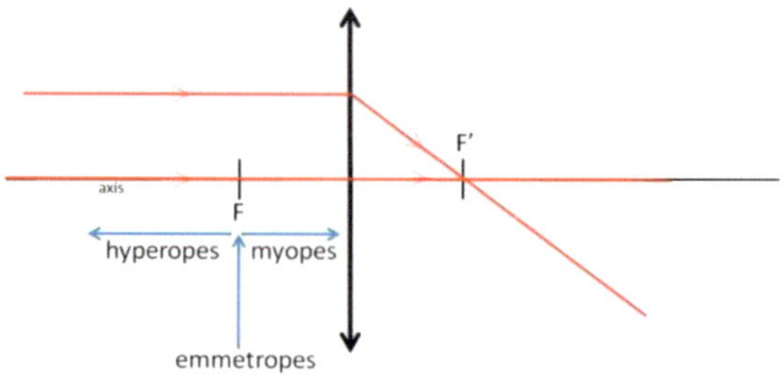


**Figure 91 The optometer principle**

Near-sighted people (myopes) need to have DIVERGING rays entering their eye in order to see distant objects clearly, and far-sighted people (hyperopes) need to have CONVERGING rays entering their eye to see distant objects clearly. As we went through this sequence of slides, you saw that, by changing the position of the object relative to F of a plus lens, you can get varying amounts of convergence or divergence of light rays. If a person who needs lenses to see clearly looks through the plus lens, he or she can find a position of the object which will allow them to measure exactly how far-sighted or near-sighted they are. People who don't need lenses to see clearly (emmetropes) will choose to put the target at F, as they are happy with parallel bundles of rays entering their eyes. Hyperopes will choose target positions outside F, while myopes will choose positions inside F.

## A PLUS LENS WITH A DIFFERENT MEDIUM ON EACH SIDE

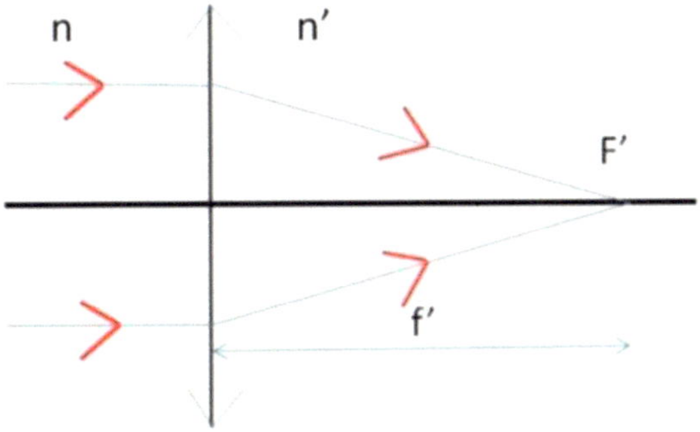


Figure 92 Considering optics of the eye

Here is a plus lens which brings rays of light from a distant object to focus at the point F', its focal point. The unit of focal power is the diopter (D). The focal power of the lens (F) = n'/f ', where n' is the refractive index of the medium on the side of F', and f ' is the focal length of the lens in meters. The refractive index of air = 1; so for a +1 diopter lens in air, the focal length is 1 meter. If we used the lens to represent the total focal power of the eye, and knew that the length of the eyeball was 22 millimeters, and that the refractive index of the eye's contents (n') was 1.33, then the optimal focal power of the eye would be 1.33/.022 = +60.5 diopters.

## THE EYE'S OPTICAL SYSTEM

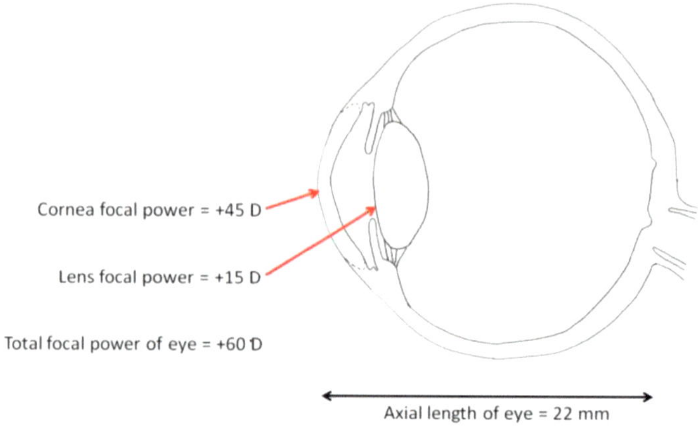


**Figure 93 Optical components of the eye**

Here is a look at the eye's optical system. The cornea is highly curved, and there is a significant difference between the refractive index of air on the one side and the corneal tissue on the other. As a result, the focal power of the cornea is high: about +45 diopters (D). The lens of the eye, although it has two surfaces with fairly high curvatures, is surrounded by aqueous humor on one side and vitreous humor on the other. The refractive index difference for rays entering and leaving the lens is comparatively small, and the focal power of the lens is considerably less than that of the cornea.

As mentioned earlier, the axial length of the eye (which can be easily measured using ultrasound) is well-suited to its optical power. Whether or not a distant object is imaged sharply on the retina depends on the balance of many factors: corneal power, crystalline lens power, crystalline lens location, and axial length. If, for example, the axial length were 20 mm, and the focal power of the eye +60 D, then using the formula from Figure 92, the optimal power would be +66.5 D, and the person would need to wear a +6.5 D lens to see clearly. An axial length of 24 mm would necessitate wearing a -5.5 D lens to see clearly. Without wearing a correction for this degree of short-sightedness, the visual acuity would be 20/140, far less than the usual 20/50 requirement for driving.

The focal power of a surface like the cornea = (n'-n)/r, where n' is the refractive index of the cornea, n is the refractive index of air, and r is the radius of curvature of the cornea, in meters. The refractive index of the cornea is 1.3375 and that of air is 1.00. Knowing the power of the cornea to be +45 D, we can calculate that the radius of curvature of the cornea is 7.5 millimeters--a pretty high curvature.

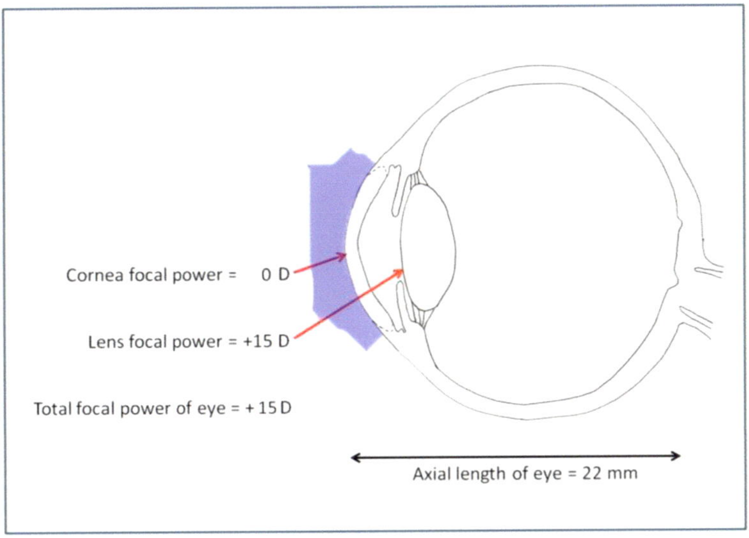


Figure 94 The eye in water is greatly underpowered

If the eye is immersed in water, then bending of light by the cornea does not happen (the cornea has a refractive index very close to that of water). This means that the eye is underpowered by 45 diopters, which means that the image of distant objects will fall way behind the retina. A child can increase the power of the crystalline lens by 10 D (an adult can do much less), so nobody will be able to see clearly under water. The remedy for this would be to put on a swim goggle or mask, which will place air once again in front of the cornea so it can become a refracting surface again. Many people have had correcting lenses mounted inside their swim masks, so that any focus problems they have when out of the water can be corrected while under water. Although fish have a cornea, it has never had any focal power. The lenses of fish developed to provide all of the focal power for their eyes, and are nearly spherical.

# Chapter 7 COMMON EYE PROBLEMS

## BLURRY DISTANCE VISION

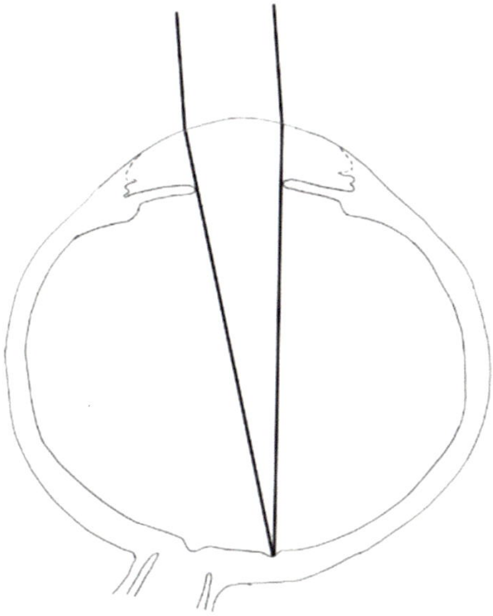

Figure 95 Emmetropic eye

This person has an in-focus image on the fovea: no problem! (To more easily show the way light rays travel into the eye in cases of refractive error, the following sequence of images represents all of the power of the eye as being at the front, which is why the corneal thickness and the crystalline lens are omitted in these diagrams. Obviously, in reality, the rays are bent as they pass through the cornea and the crystalline lens.) The rays entering the eye are parallel to each other, as they are coming from a distant point source of light, such as a star. If an eye, in its relaxed state (more about that shortly) can receive an in-focus image of a distant object, it is said to be emmetropic.

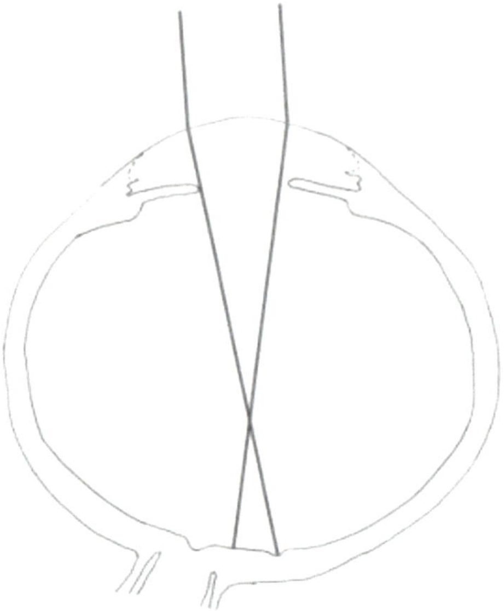

Figure 96 Myopic eye

This eye has a focal power which is too high: light from a distant object is focused at a point ahead of the retina; therefore, the distant object will be seen blurred. It is said to be near-sighted or myopic. The word comes from the Greek, ‘to squint’, which is what near-sighted people sometimes do in order to decrease the blur of images. If this person moved closer to the object they were looking at, the image would move back toward the retina, which is why myopic people are called 'near-sighted'--they can see better when they are at a shorter distance from the objects they are looking at.

There are various reasons why an eye is overpowered: the eyeball may be longer than necessary, or the optical system may be more powerful than necessary, or a combination of both.

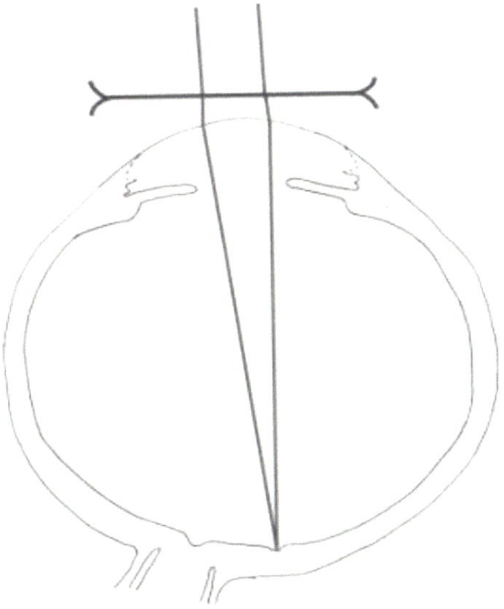

**Figure 97  Correction of myopia**

To correct the vision of a near-sighted person, a minus lens is placed in front of the eye. The desired correcting lens will diverge the parallel rays which strike it (shown at the top, just before the rays enter the eye) enough to overcome the overly-strong refractive power of the eye, causing the rays to come to a focus at the retina, making the distant object seen clearly.

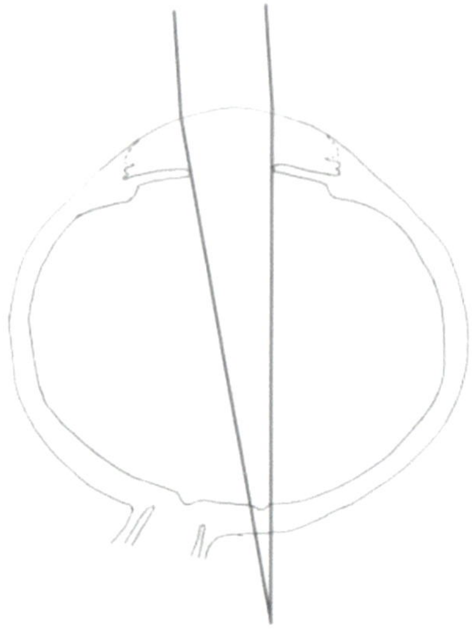

Figure 98 Hyperopic eye

For a far-sighted eye, the image of a distant object falls behind the retina, therefore it will be seen blurred. The focal power of this eye is less than required to bring the image to a focus at the fovea. If this person moves closer to the object they are looking at, the image will move farther behind the retina, and it will be even more blurry. The person will prefer to keep objects they are looking at as far away as possible, which is why people with this focusing problem are referred to as 'far-sighted' or hyperopic—they see far away objects clearer than they see nearby objects. People under the age of 60 have the ability to increase the focal power of their eye (called accommodation) to some degree. If this person is only somewhat far-sighted, they could clear up the image of a distant object by using accommodation to increase the focal power of the eye. If they look at a nearby object, they must further increase the focal power of the eye. This work may cause eyestrain.

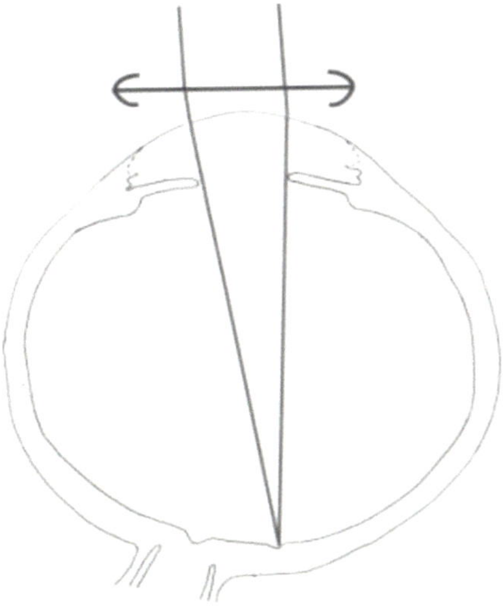

Figure 99  Correction of hyperopia

There are various reasons why an eye is underpowered:  the eyeball may be shorter than necessary, or the optical system may be less powerful than necessary, or a combination of both.

A plus (converging) lens will bring the focal point up to the retina, so the distant object is seen clearly.  People with a small hyperopic refractive error may use accommodation to clear up distance vision.  Using a plus lens in these cases will also allow the eye to relax when looking at distant objects because accommodation will not be required to see distant objects clearly.

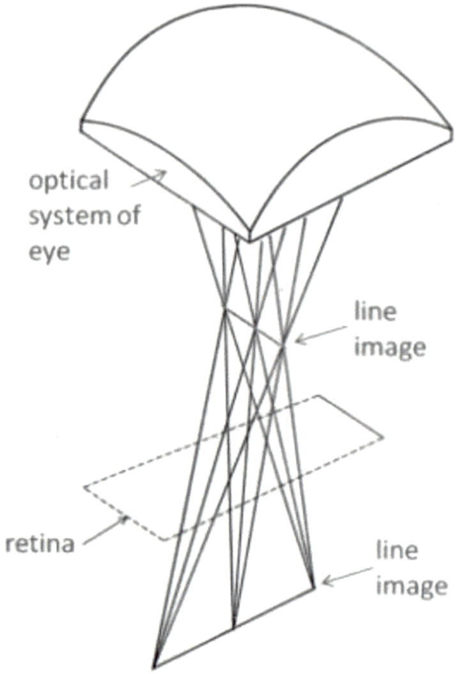


Figure 100 Astigmatism

The previous examples were for eyes which had the same focal power in all directions. Such systems are called spherical. Eyes with a spherical optical system have a refracting system shaped like a basketball: if you make a slice through the center of a basketball, the curvature of the system will be the same wherever you slice. In the case of astigmatism, the eye has a refracting system shaped like a football: slices through the center of a football will give you different curvatures depending on the direction of the slice. The word 'astigmatism' means that the eye is not capable of producing a point image for a point object: in fact the eye produces TWO line images for each single point object being looked at. People with astigmatism may notice double images of objects they are looking at with one eye. The line images both could be ahead of the retina, or both behind the retina, or on either side of the retina as shown here. The position of these line images relative to the retina depends on the overall power of the eye. Most people have a small degree of astigmatism.

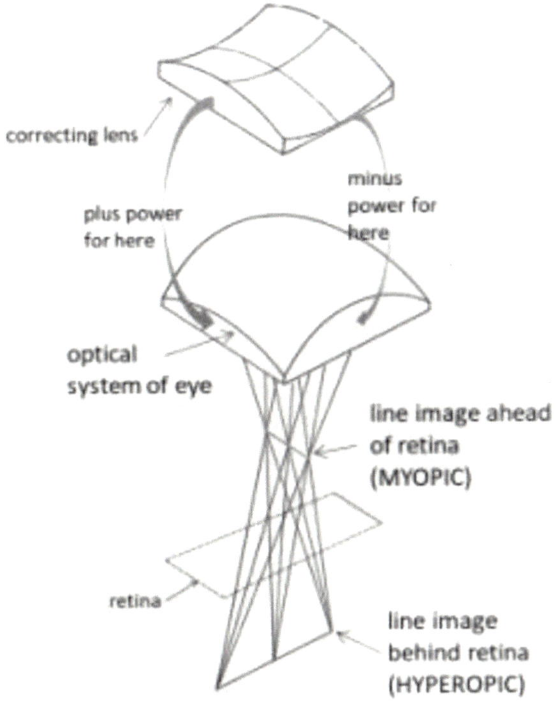


Figure 101 Correcting astigmatism

Figure 101 shows a correcting lens for astigmatism. Note that one of the two line images falls ahead of the retina: this part of the system is overpowered (myopic). The other line image falls behind the retina: this part of the system is underpowered (hyperopic). The correcting lens will need plus power in one direction and minus power in the other.

A lens with different powers in different directions is called a toric or cylindrical lens. As the correct lens powers are gradually added, the two line foci will each get shorter, and will come closer together, until (with the correct toric lens in place), the two line foci collapse into a single point image on the retina. The system is now stigmatic: a point object will give rise to a point image.

The correcting lens must be correctly oriented: if (for example) a spectacle frame gets bent so that the lenses are rotated, the vision will be worse. The standard notation for a spectacle lens prescription includes: (1) power of the spherical lens required, (2) power of the cylindrical lens required, (3) the axis or orientation of the cylindrical lens required. A person with a spherical refractive error will have parts (2) and (3) of the prescription blank. A person with astigmatism will have all three parts filled in. For the sake of discussion, let's say that the line image ahead of the retina is vertical and the line image behind the retina is horizontal. Let's say further that each line image is 1 millimeter from the retina. In terms of focal power, this 1 millimeter discrepancy is equivalent to 3 diopters for each line image. The distance between the two line foci is 2 millimeters: this means the amount of astigmatism for this eye is 6 diopters.

A spherical correcting lens of +3.00 would have this focal power in all directions. It would pull the hyperopic line image up to the retina, but would also move the myopic line image 6 diopters farther away from the retina: so the cylindrical part of the correction would need to be -6.00 D in order to move the myopic line image back to the retina. This prescription would be written: +3.00 -6.00 x 90. It could also be written -3.00 +6.00 x 180.

The confusing part of this discussion is that for a cylindrical lens, the axis is the direction in which it has no focal power. The lens prescription is actually describing the power and orientation of two lenses combined: a spherical lens and a cylindrical lens. The spherical lens has the same dioptric power in all directions, while the cylindrical lens only has its full power at right angles to the cylinder axis, and no power along its axis. A lens specified as +3.00 -6.00 x 90 is referred to as a sphero-cylindrical lens: you could consider it as a spherical lens with +3.00 diopters in all directions, combined with a cylindrical lens which would be written as 0.00 -6.00 x 90.

## NORMAL BINOCULAR VISION

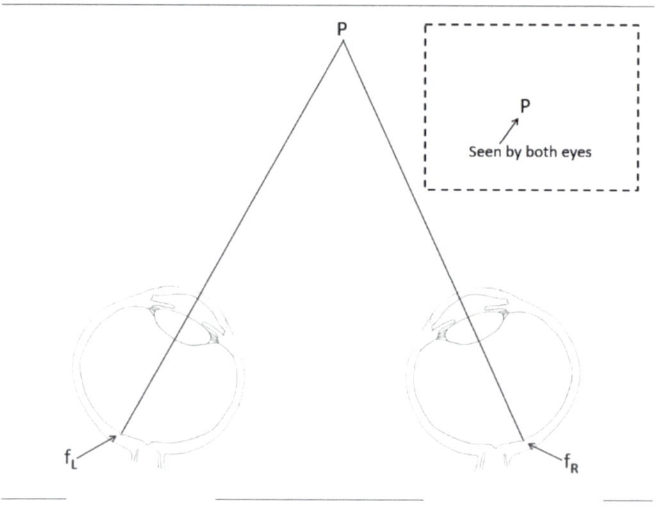


Figure 102  Normal binocular vision

Having normal binocular vision is a remarkable accomplishment: each eye is moved by six different muscles, and those six muscles are controlled by three separate cranial nerves. To have both eyes look accurately at the same point requires successful co-operation of twelve muscles and six cranial nerves. If everything works correctly, an image of the point P will fall on each fovea. In Figure 102, a person with normal binocular vision is looking at the point P. The fovea of the left eye ($f_L$) and the fovea of the right eye ($f_R$) are lined up with the point P.

The two foveas are described as corresponding points: an object which is imaged on each fovea will stimulate the same location in the visual cortex, and will be seen in the same direction. Images provided by both foveas will be seen as a single object. The box enclosed by dashes represents the VISUAL WORLD, while the rest of the diagram represents the PHYSICAL WORLD. The merging of the two images also allows the brain to detect small differences between them (after all, there is a distance of some 6 centimeters between the two viewpoints, so there will be some differences). These small differences are used by the brain to build up a three-dimensional impression of the world called stereopsis.

If there are small errors in alignment of the eyes, these may be compensated for by increased muscle activity, in order to maintain correct position of the two foveas. In some cases, increased muscle activity may lead to eyestrain. Because the muscles which move the eyes are voluntary muscles, they may benefit from eye exercises, so that the eyestrain can be reduced.

## DOUBLE VISION

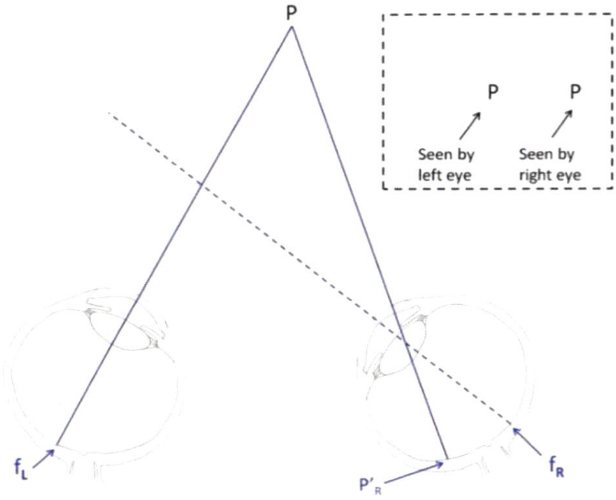


**Figure 103 Esotropia causes double vision**

Eye alignment problems can occur in many directions (because of muscle problems or neurological problems): there are many different types of *strabismus*. The misaligned eye may be looking too far upward, downward, inward, or outward. When there is an outward turned eye, the condition would be termed *exotropia*.

This person is able to look accurately at the point P with the left eye only: the image falls on the left fovea and is seen straight ahead as shown in the VISUAL WORLD box. For this example, the person has esotropia. The right eye is turned inward.

In Fig. 103, the right eye is not able to aim its fovea correctly at the point P. The image of P will not land on the fovea of the right eye, but at the position $P'_R$. The image of P for the right eye will not be seen in the same direction as the image of P for the left eye. In this situation, the person will see the point doubled. For the left eye, the image will be straight ahead, while the doubled image seen by the right eye will be to the right of the first image. The reason for this location is that, for the right eye, the image is falling on retina nasal to the fovea, so the image will be perceived as lying to the right of the straight-ahead position, and to the right of the image of P provided by the left eye.

Seeing double poses problems, as the person must decide which image to pay attention to--which doorway to walk through, for example. As a result, over time, the brain may begin to ignore the wrong image, and may tune it out altogether, resulting in amblyopia (lazy eye). If strabismus is present at birth, the vision of the turned eye may not develop to its full potential.

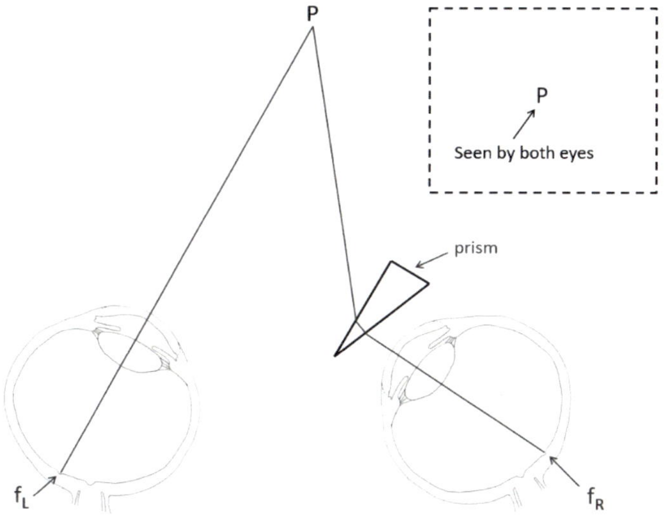


Figure 104 Correcting double vision of esotrope

To correct esotropia, a prism placed before the right eye allows the image of P to land on the right fovea. This prism is described as a 'relieving prism' as it allows the right eye to remain in its turned position, yet allows the image to fall on the right fovea. This will eliminate the double vision, and the person will see a single object P straight ahead in their visual world.

## COLOR BLINDNESS

To talk about problems with color vision, we must first take a look at the opsins in the cones (see Figure 49). Cones whose opsin absorbs energy mainly in the red portion of the spectrum may be referred to as RED CONES. Similarly, we have GREEN CONES and BLUE CONES. One in 12 men inherit a defective gene, resulting in some form of color vision defect due to synthesis of a defective opsin. One in 200 women have the same problem. The defective gene results in a defective opsin protein in cones. People with color vision defects should avoid training for vocations where color judgement is critical, such as electronics and operating aircraft.

The visible spectrum of light extends from violet to red, that is, from wavelength of 400 nanometers to 700 nanometers. Surprisingly, the normal numbers of red, green, and blue cones are not even close to equal: there are more red ones (about 55% of cones) than green ones (about 40% of cones), while the blue cones are a low 5% of cones. Unless a person is born with NO cones, they will see color, although differently than the average person. If there is a problem with the red cones, the person will have problems seeing red: if the defect is mild, the term is protanomaly. If there are no red cones, the term is protanopia. Parallel terms are used for people who have problems with green cones: deuteranomaly and deuteranopia. Problems with blue cones are a logical possibility, but rare. The terms in this case are tritanomaly and tritanopia.

Because the genes which code for color vision are on the X chromosome, women with their double X chromosome are ten times less likely than men to inherit a color vision defect. The extra X chromosome in women can compensate for a defect on one X chromosome. As men have only one X chromosome (being XY), they cannot overcome a defect in the X chromosome if one is present.

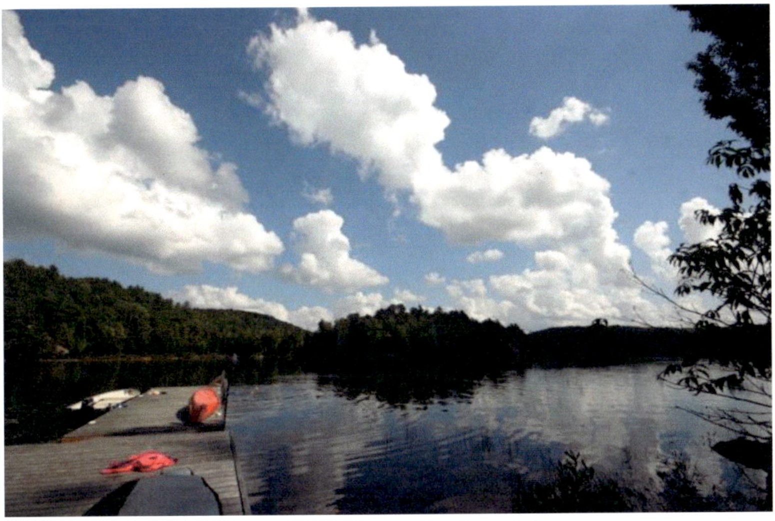

Figure 105 Normal color vision

Here is a scene as it would be perceived by a person with a normal balance of red, green, and blue cones. The canoe is red, the trees in the distance are green, and the sky is blue.

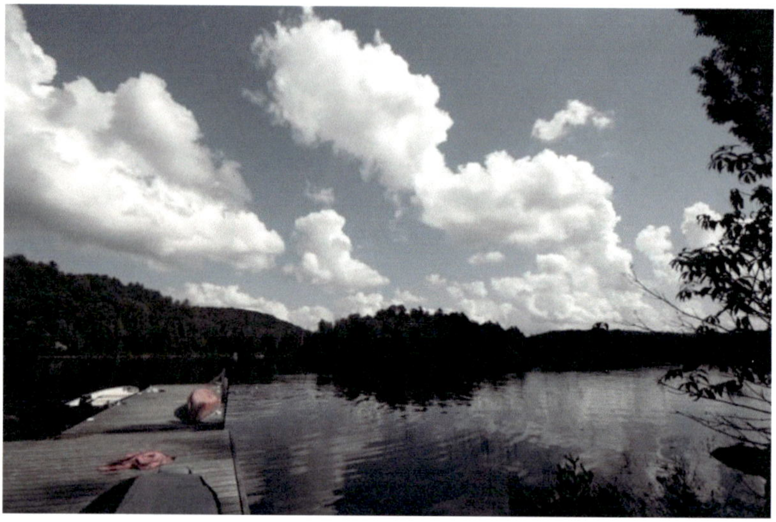

Figure 106  Image simulates red cone deficiency

Here is a simulation of what the previous scene might look like to a person with a deficiency in red cones. The canoe is not very red. The rest of the colors appear paler. Perception, of course, is a very personal thing: if a person has seen the same way all their life, they may not be aware of the differences in their own perception.

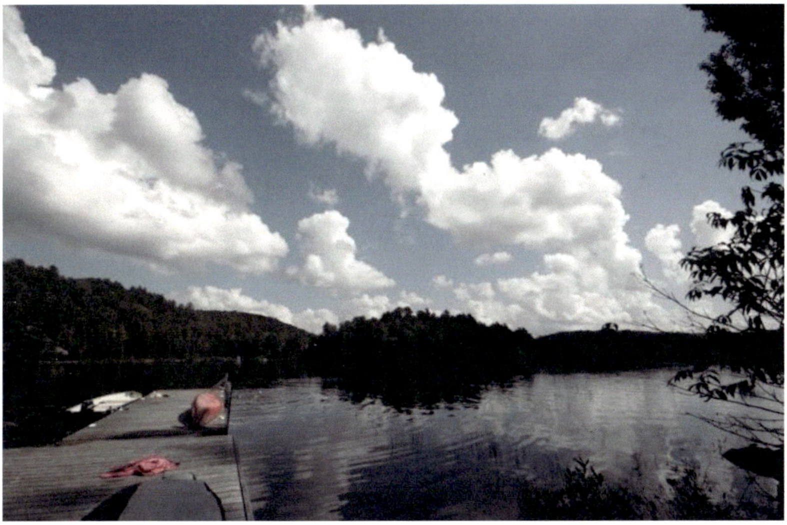

**Figure 107  Image simulates green cone deficiency**

Here is an attempt to show what might be seen by a person with a deficiency in green cones. The trees in the distance are less green. Again, most colors appear paler.

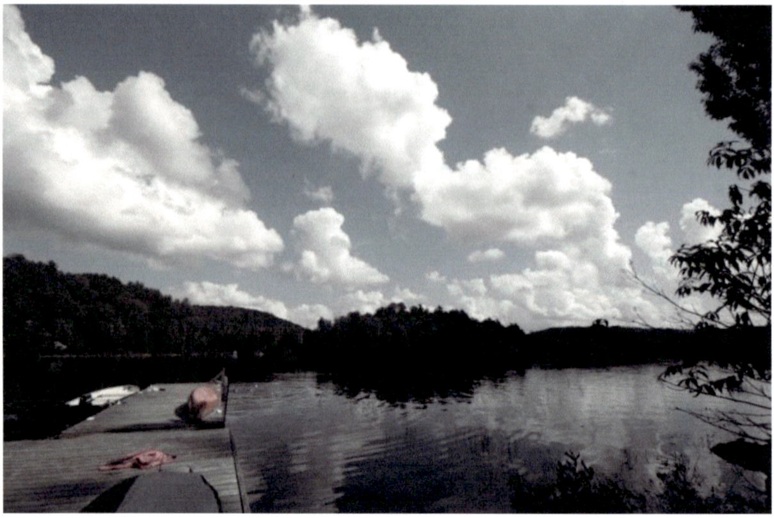

Figure 108  Image simulates blue cone deficiency

Here is a rendering of what the scene might look like to a person with a deficiency of blue cones. The sky is definitely not blue, but the other colors are also paler.

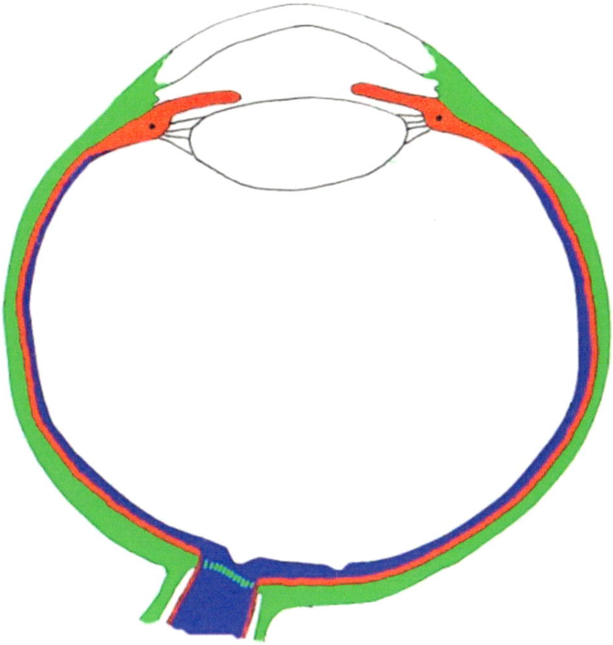

Figure 109 Normal color vision

A normal view of the layer diagrams from this book, as seen by a person with a normal population of red, green, and blue cones.

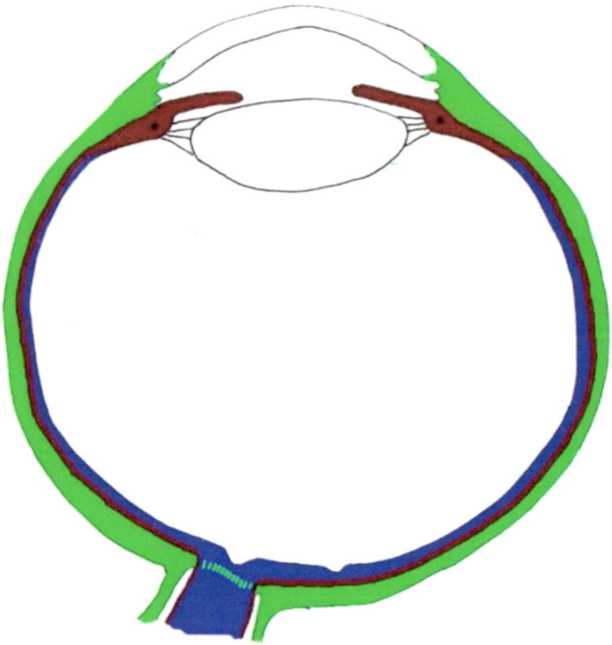

Figure 110  Red cone deficiency

Here is a somewhat exaggerated example of what the diagram would look like to a person with a red cone deficiency.

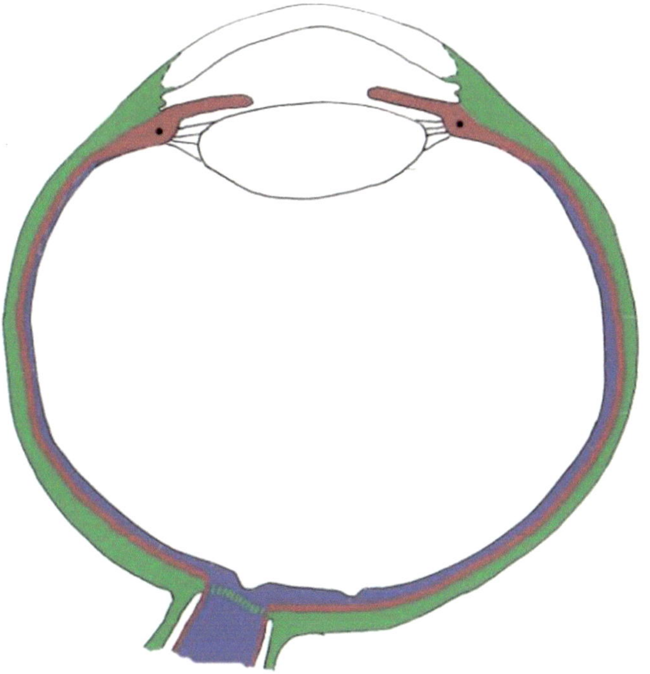

Figure 111 Green cone deficiency

A person with a deficiency of green cones would see the diagram like this. Note particularly that the difference between red and green is not as marked as in Fig. 109.

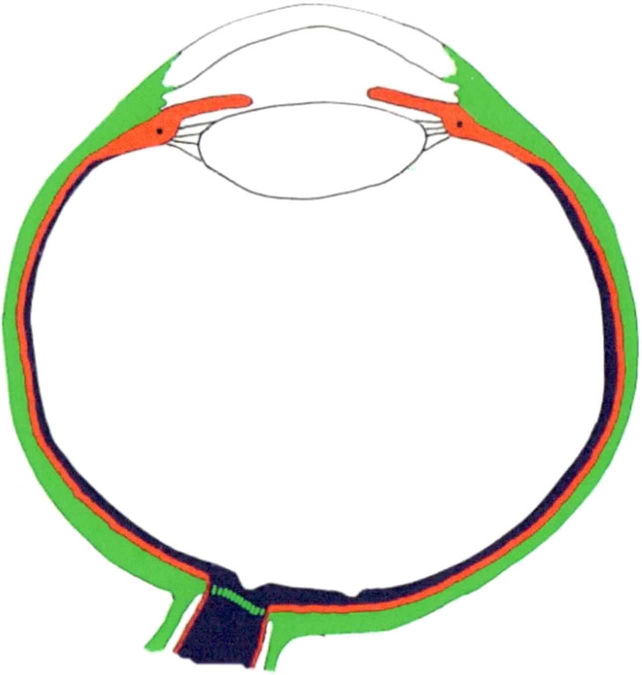

Figure 112 Blue cone deficiency

A person with a deficiency in blue cones would have a view like this and find the blue hard to distinguish from black.

# VISUAL FIELD

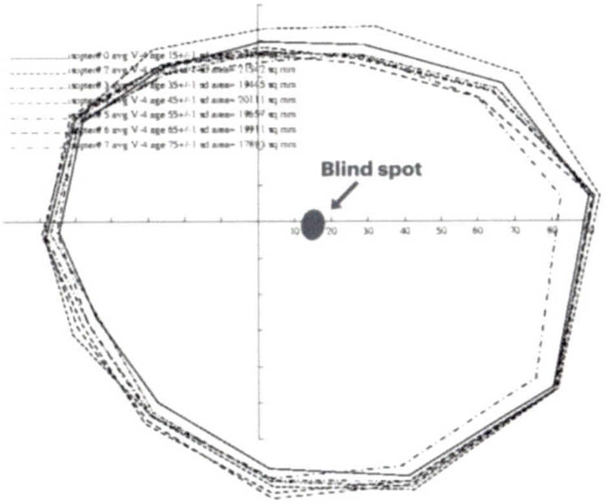


Figure 113 Normal Visual Field for **ages 15 - 75**

## Visual Field Testing

The visual field is the area within which a spot of light of specified size and brightness can be seen. Because of the structure of the eye, the visual field also normally contains a blindspot, which is usually about 5 degrees wide x 7 degrees high, with its center 15 degrees temporal from the fixation point: that is, 15 degrees to the right of the fixation point for the right eye. (By the way, the blindspot was first studied by the French physicist Mariotte in 1668).

In order to measure a visual field, the patient is seated before an instrument (a perimeter), one eye is covered, and the patient is required to maintain a steady gaze on an object straight ahead (the fixation point). This is where the test becomes difficult: a spot is moved from a position where you cannot see it, and you are asked to report when you see it, but you are asked NOT to look at it. If that isn't bad enough, you also need to accept a <u>fair amount of</u>

uncertainty: you should respond when you THINK you see the spot, and not wait until you are CERTAIN you saw the spot. This is because a field test is trying to locate the THRESHOLD, a point between an area where you are sure you CAN'T see the spot and an area where you are sure you CAN see the spot. When the spot is ON the threshold, then 50% of the time you think you can see it, and 50% of the time you think you can't see it. To find the outer limit of the visual field, the spot starts moving from the extreme periphery; to find the limits of the blind spot, the test spot is placed inside the blind spot area and moved outward.

The fields shown in Figure 113 were obtained with a large, bright test spot. The outer limit of the field is smaller for more difficult test spots, and the blind spot becomes larger for more difficult test spots. There are various perimeters in use, many of them automated, and some manual. Although the field becomes smaller with age, the size of the field for the 75 year old group is still large enough to meet the standard for driving. Note that the inferior temporal field is the largest, while the superior nasal field is the smallest. Since we are terrestrial creatures, we are more interested in details in our lower field of vision. With both eyes open, our visual fields are well able to let us know about objects or threats coming from the sides.

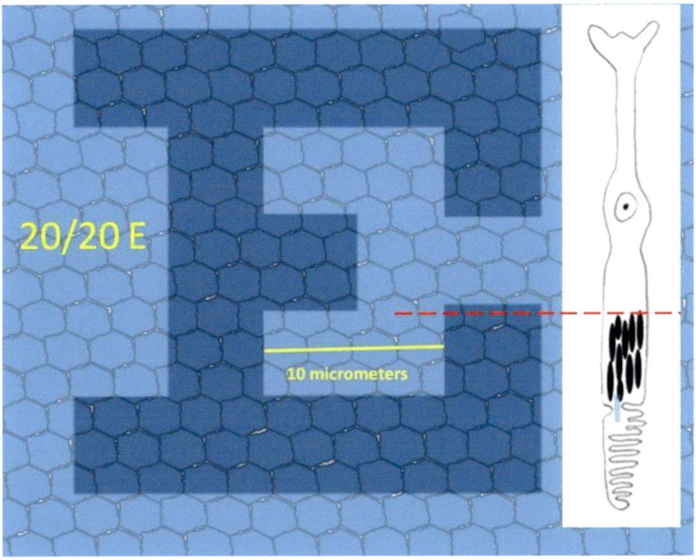


Figure 114 20/20 E on cone mosaic

The spacing of cones in the fovea was studied by Christine Curcio and co-workers (Journal of Comparative Neurology 1990;292:497).

The 20/20 E lands on a matrix of 10 x 10 foveal cones. The cones are about 2.5 micrometers in width (a human hair is 80 micrometers wide). The image of the 20/20 E on the retina is 25 x 25 micrometers. Before anything can appear in the visual field, it must stimulate the retina, so this is where it all begins. The dashed red line in this image shows the level of the retina at which this matrix is readily seen in a microscope. Images taken more toward the bottom of the cone (the outer segment) are more variable and harder to interpret.

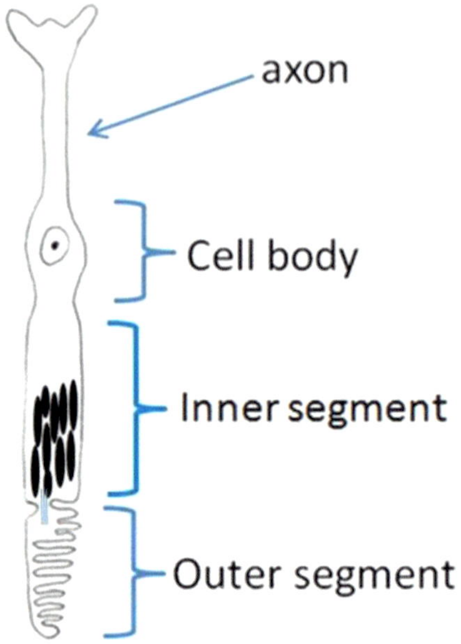


**Figure 115 Cone by itself**

Here is a single foveal cone, all by itself. It is the first player in the visual process. The process of vision is triggered by absorption of light in photopigment in the outer segment of the receptor. This causes a change in the membrane of the cell which is transmitted via the axon to the next player in the visual pathway, the bipolar cell. The black objects in the inner segment are mitochondria which supply energy for making new photopigment and for transmitting impulses to the axon. The inner and outer segments of the photoreceptors pass through the external limiting membrane of the retina, while the rest of the photoreceptor is within the retina (that is, between the external and internal limiting membranes of the retina).

When Curcio and her team were using the microscope to examine the pattern formed by photoreceptors, they found that the best level to get a sense of the pattern was to focus at the level about midway through the inner segment (shown by a red line in the previous image). The outer segments were too fine and wavy to get a sense of the pattern of photoreceptors.

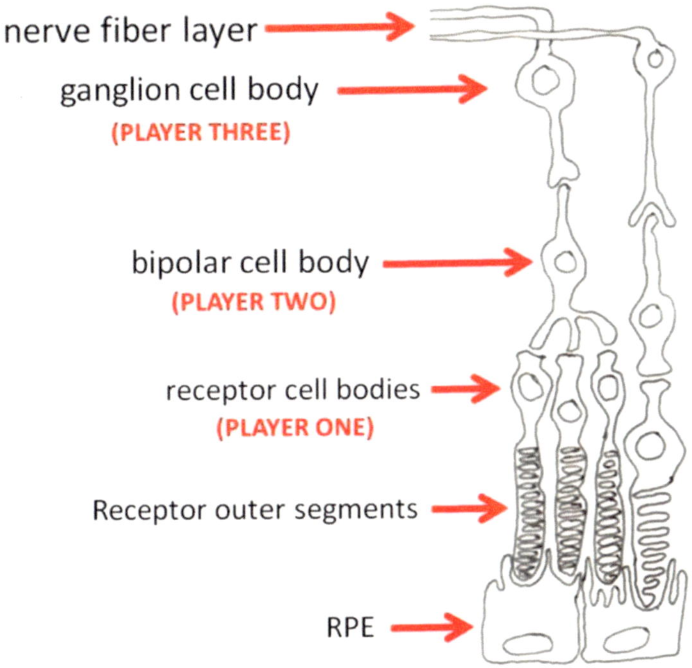


Figure 116 Retinal players in visual process

## The retinal players in sending visual information to the brain

When the photoreceptors (rods and cones are shown at the bottom of the figure) are stimulated, they pass on that stimulation to the next two retinal players in the visual process, the bipolar cell and ganglion cell. The ganglion cell passes on visual impulses along its axons in the nerve fiber layer of the retina, which continue all the way to the fourth player, the optic radiation cell, in the lateral geniculate body in the middle of the brain. Nerve fibers are not just wires carrying electrical impulses: they are part of living cells (neurons). There is a steady traffic of material moving via axoplasmic flow to and from the cell body of ganglion cells. If there is an interruption in the function of a Ganglion Cell Axon at a point in the retina, say due to diabetes or hypertension for example, material travelling via axoplasmic flow may be seen accumulating in the retina at the location of the damage.

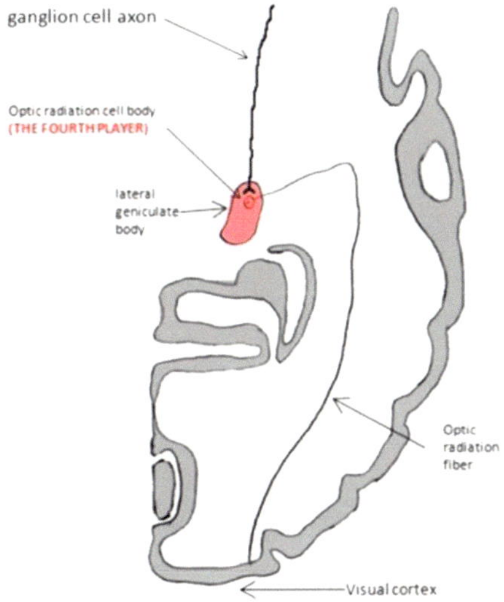


Figure 117 Player 4 in lateral geniculate body

## The fourth player in the visual process

The path from the lateral geniculate body to the visual cortex.

Here is a horizontal section through the midbrain. After its long travel from the retina, the axon of the retinal ganglion cell connects with the fourth player in the visual process, the optic radiation cell, whose cell body is in the lateral geniculate body. From there, the axon of the optic radiation cell travels to the visual cortex, where the news from the retina begins its processing into visual information.

# VISUAL FIELD LOSS

## PROBLEMS CLOSE TO THE EYE

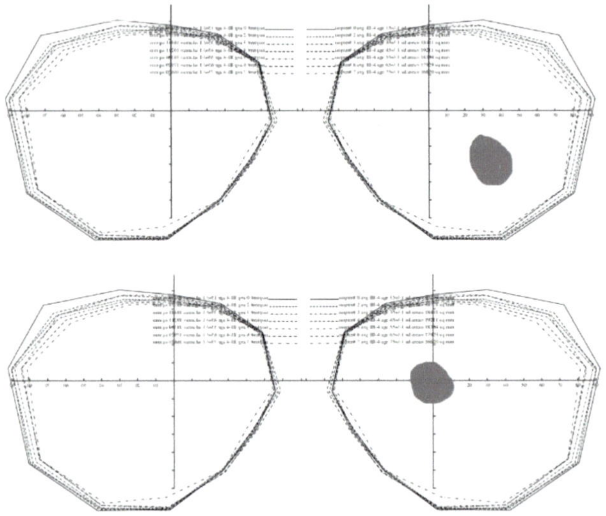

Figure 118 Field losses due to damage close to eye

Gray areas show potential field losses caused by retinal problems (upper figure of Figure 118) or optic nerve problems (lower figure). The nerves carrying visual information travel along the visual pathway. Until they reach the chiasm (the point where about half of the Ganglion Cell Axons cross over to the other side of the brain), the axons from each eye travel separately. When visual field loss is found for one eye only, the problem must lie somewhere ahead of the chiasm. In the case of retinal damage, for example caused by infection, trauma, or retinal detachment, the field loss will be in one visual field only. For the upper example, the damaged retina must be in the right eye, and superior and nasal to the foveal center, because the right visual field loss is inferior and temporal to the fixation point (the central point of the field).

In the lower example, a typical field loss due to damage to the right optic nerve is shown. Because axons from the foveal region occupy a large portion of the optic nerve, it is likely that the field loss caused by a problem with the right optic nerve (optic neuritis due to multiple sclerosis, for example) will affect the very center of the visual field. The field loss shown in the lower figure could, of course, also be due to retinal damage in the right eye, involving the fovea.

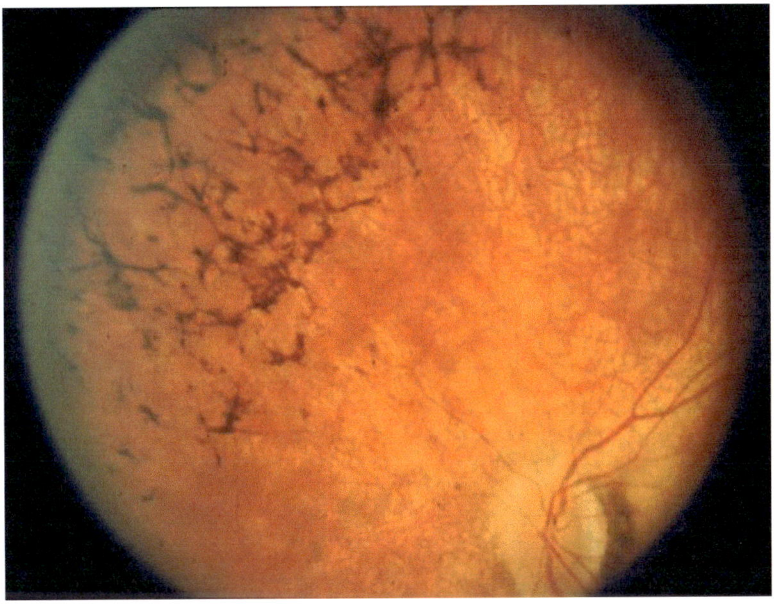

**Figure 119 Retinitis pigmentosa**

Here is a view of the superior nasal periphery of the left eye for a patient with retinitis pigmentosa (RP). For this person, both eyes showed the black cobwebby appearance all around the clock in the peripheral retina. Retinitis pigmentosa is an inherited condition in which the photoreceptors and retinal pigment epithelium (RPE) of both eyes slowly degenerate. When the RPE cells fail, they release their black pigment granules as seen here.

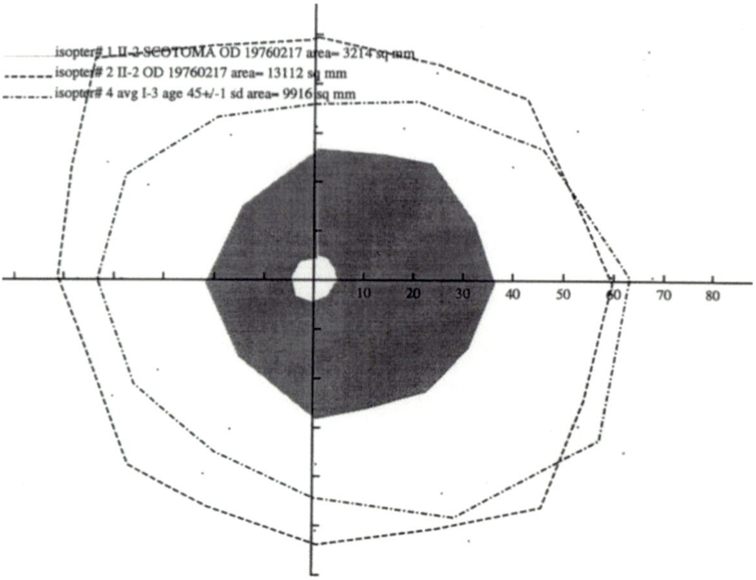


**Figure 120 Field loss in retinitis pigmentosa**

Here is the visual field for one eye of a person with retinitis pigmentosa. The other eye had similar results. Although field losses may vary, the presence of a 'ring scotoma' such as shown here is fairly common. This person has a visual field which was working fine for the central ten degrees, but outside that there is a non-seeing area (scotoma). Outside the ring scotoma, the peripheral field is normal. When this person tried to catch a ball tossed to her, she could see the ball as it was thrown, using her peripheral vision, but then it would enter the non-seeing area. By the time she could see it in the central part of her field, it was very difficult to catch.

## PROBLEMS NEAR THE CHIASM

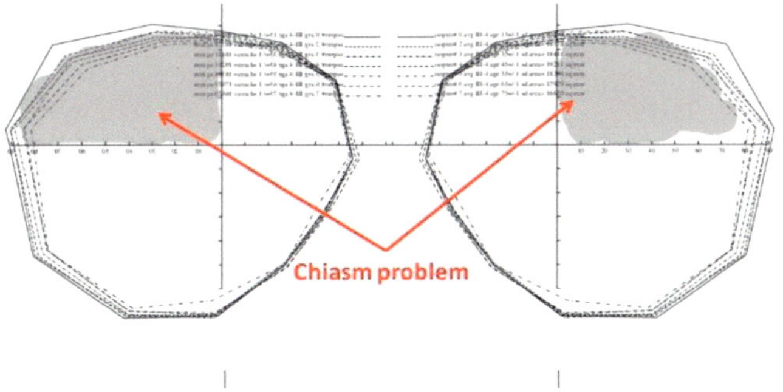


**Figure 121 Field losses due to pressure on underside of chiasm from pituitary tumor**

At the center of the chiasm, there is a great gathering of Ganglion Cell Axons which are crossing from opposite sides of the visual pathway. For each eye, the axons from the nasal retina cross at the center of the chiasm. Because the pituitary gland lies just below the chiasm, a problem such as a pituitary tumor may cause pressure on the underside of the chiasm.

Axons which cross at the lower part of the chiasm are serving the lower nasal retina of each eye: the tumor may cause a field loss for the superior temporal field of each eye. This is shown in Figure 121. Field losses are on opposite sides of the visual fields.

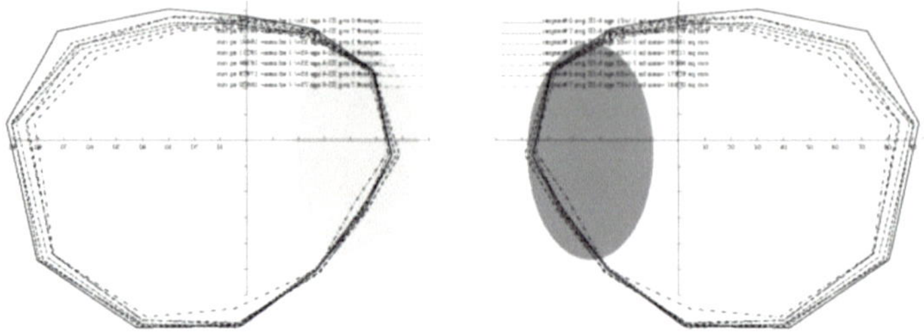

Figure 122 Field losses due to aneurysm of right internal carotid

Here is the sort of visual field disturbance which would be associated with aneurysm of the right internal carotid artery adjacent to the chiasm. The major impact of the enlargement of the internal carotid artery would be on the ganglion cell axons on the right side of the chiasm. These are the non-crossing fibres from the temporal retina of the right eye. This would result in a disturbance in the nasal visual field of the right eye (darkened area). As the aneurysm continues to enlarge, it may push the chiasm sideways toward the left, where it may start to press itself against the left internal carotid artery, affecting the non-crossing axons from the left eye. As this pressure is likely to be less than that on the right side of the chiasm, the nasal field disturbance for the left eye will be less marked (less darkened area shown in Figure 122).

## PROBLEMS AFTER THE CHIASM (closer to the visual cortex)

After the chiasm, the Ganglion Cell Axons reach the lateral geniculate body, where they connect with the fourth player in the visual pathway, the optic radiation cell. By the time they reach the lateral geniculate body, axons from corresponding parts of the retina are travelling together.

Damage in these higher parts of the visual pathway will result in visual field loss on the same side of the visual fields.

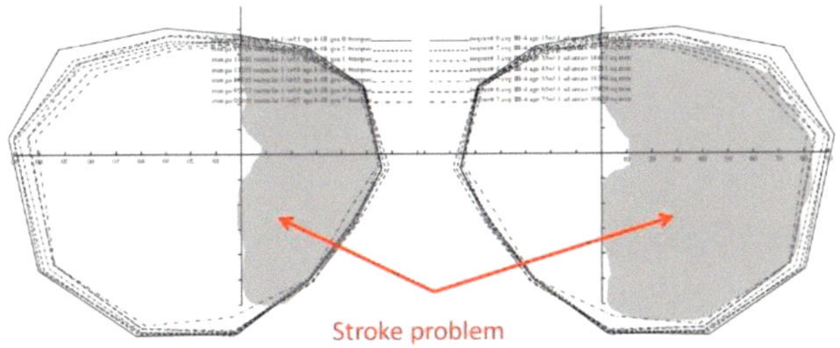


**Figure 123 Field loss due to stroke involving left visual cortex**

Figure 123 shows the visual field loss resulting from a stroke affecting the visual cortex on the left side of the brain: vision to the person's right is lost. Because a large portion of the visual cortex is dedicated to vision from the foveal regions, often some of the central vision is still working. This is called macular sparing.

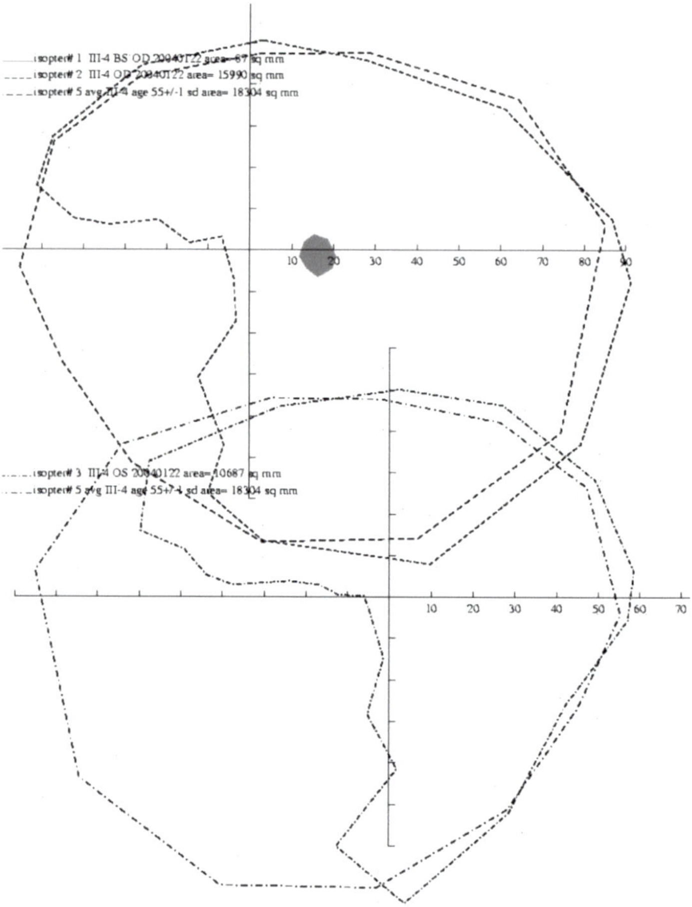


**Figure 124 Field loss due to parietal lobe tumor**

The upper part of this diagram is the field test result for the right eye, and the lower is for the left eye. This person had a tumor affecting the right parietal lobe of the brain. For each part, a field norm is superimposed on the person's test result. You can see that there is disturbance to the field to the left for each eye. The lower left part of each field is much smaller than normal. As the upper optic radiations move from the lateral geniculate body to the visual cortex, some of them loop upward into the parietal lobe. These fibres were damaged by a right parietal lobe tumor, resulting in the lower left field loss for each eye.

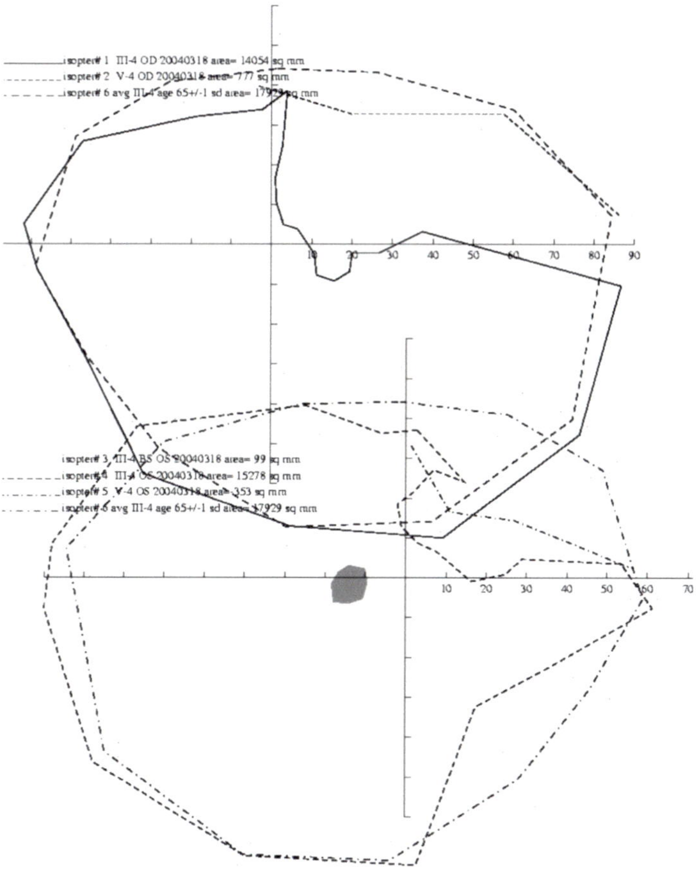


Figure 125  Field loss due temporal lobe tumor

This person had a stroke involving the temporal lobe of the brain, on the left side of the brain. The upper drawing shows the field test result for the right eye, while the upper one shows results for the left eye. The more regular pattern on the outside is a visual field norm. You will note that the field is smaller than normal to the right for each eye, and that the upper right area is more affected than the lower right. This occurs because the lower optic radiations loop into the temporal lobe on their way to the visual cortex. Damage to the left temporal lobe may cause problems in the upper right visual field. The blindspot for the left eye is normal, while it is only possible to locate the lower edge of the blindspot for the right. The field above the blindspot for the right eye falls within the non-seeing area.

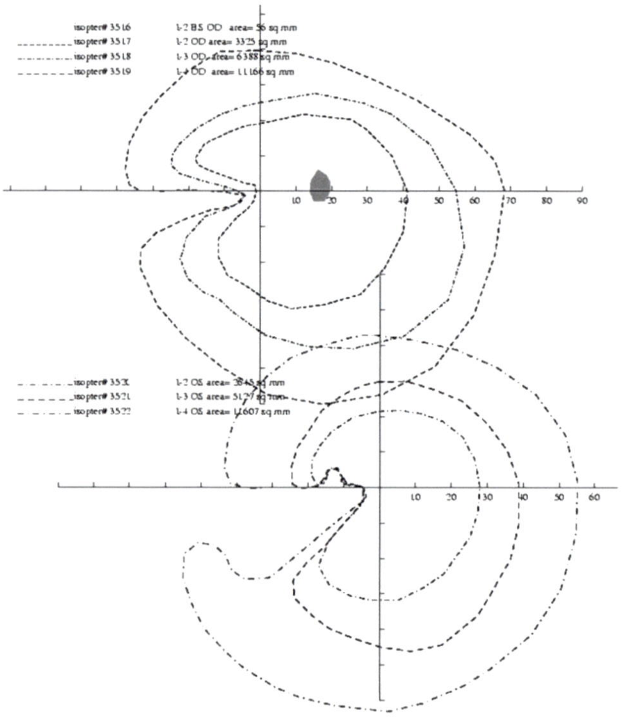


Figure 126 Field loss due to lateral geniculate body tumor

Damage to the lateral geniculate body will cause field loss for both eyes. This field loss was caused by a tumor affecting the right lateral geniculate body, so the field loss is confined to the left visual field of both eyes. Because of the organization of lateral geniculate body, the field losses will look like a finger has been poked horizontally into the visual field. The blindspot for the right eye is normal, while only the upper edge of the blindspot may be charted for the left eye: the field below the left blindspot is included within the non-seeing area.

For people with long-standing visual field loss, it is not unusual to be 'seeing things' in the non-seeing part of their visual field. This seems to be due to the brain becoming bored with seeing nothing in these areas, and filling in the blank space randomly with things such as people, flowers, or other things. Similar occurrences may follow macular degeneration.

# RETINAL DETACHMENT

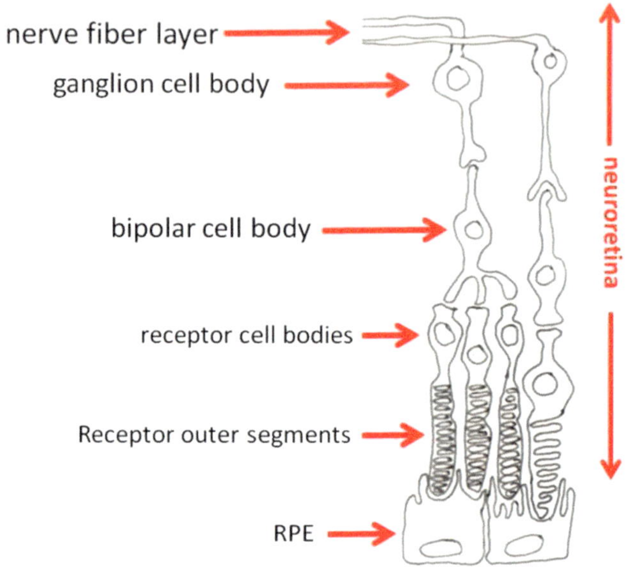


**Figure 127 Normal relation between outer segments and RPE**

Under normal conditions, the retinal pigment epithelium (RPE) closely surrounds the outer segments of the photoreceptors. During embryonic development of the retina, there is a large space between the receptor outer segments and the retinal pigment epithelium (RPE). As the eye develops, this space (the subretinal space) becomes very small, and is kept that way by the RPE, which constantly pumps fluid out of the subretinal space.

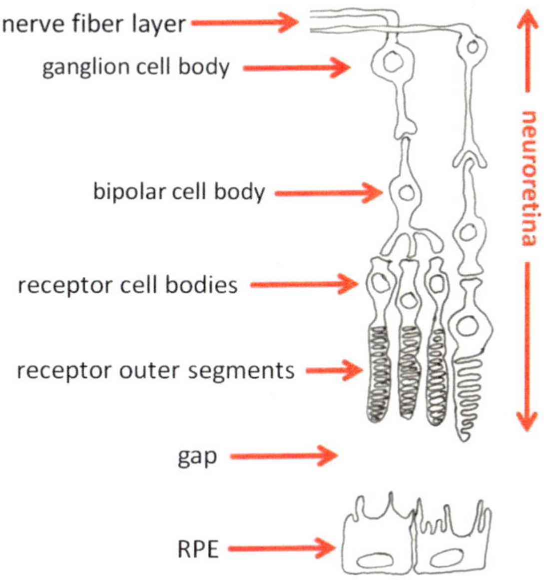


Figure 128 Gap between outer segments and RPE in retinal detachment

The neuroretina varies in thickness from 130 to 370 micrometers (a piece of paper is around 150 micrometers thick). When there is a break in the neuroretina, fluid may move into the subretinal space, creating a gap between the receptor outer segments and the retinal pigment epithelium (RPE). This is a retinal detachment. This causes some degree of impairment in the nourishment of the receptors. If the gap is small, vision in the affected area may be dimmed to some degree; if the gap is large, function of the receptors stops, and there is a non-seeing area in the visual field. Surgical correction of the retinal detachment usually involves finding the hole which allowed fluid through the retina into the subretinal space. Once that hole is closed, the RPE will gradually remove the fluid from the subretinal space, the gap will be closed, and retinal function may be restored. It's amazing what recuperative powers the eye has!

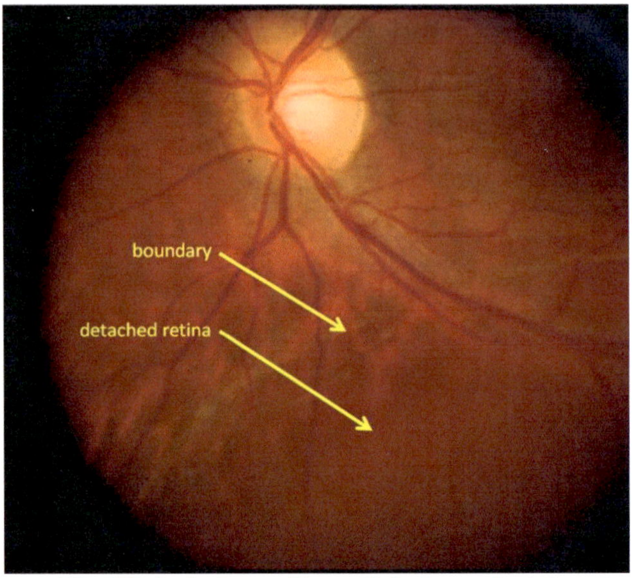


**Figure 129 Clinical photo of large inferior retinal detachemt**

Figure 129 shows a wide area of retinal detachment below the Optic Nerve Head in this left eye.

Risk factors for retinal detachment include

- congenital retinal holes
- blunt injury to the eye
- inflammations of the retina and/or choroid
- vitreous traction
- high myopia
- peripheral retinal degeneration
- cataract surgery
- Tumors under the retina may also cause detachment
- Hemorrhage caused by diabetes may also lead to retinal detachment.

The curved shape of the edge of the detachment indicates that there is a fair amount of fluid in the subretinal space. Above the boundary marked by the arrow the normally attached retina begins. Because the receptors in the lower retina have been lifted away from the retinal pigment epithelium, they are not functional, and the patient had a large non-seeing area in the superior visual field.

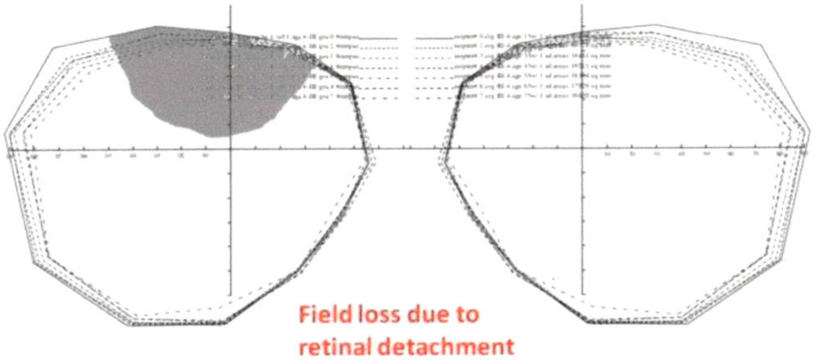


**Figure 130 Here is the visual field for the left eye of the person shown in Figure 129.**

Visual field for the left eye of the person shown in the previous image. The detached retina is in the left eye, below the foveal center. The visual field in the superior field for the left eye has a curved edge matching that of the border of the detachment, and begins about five degrees superior to the fixation point for the field (the intersection of the two straight lines on the field).

## DIABETES

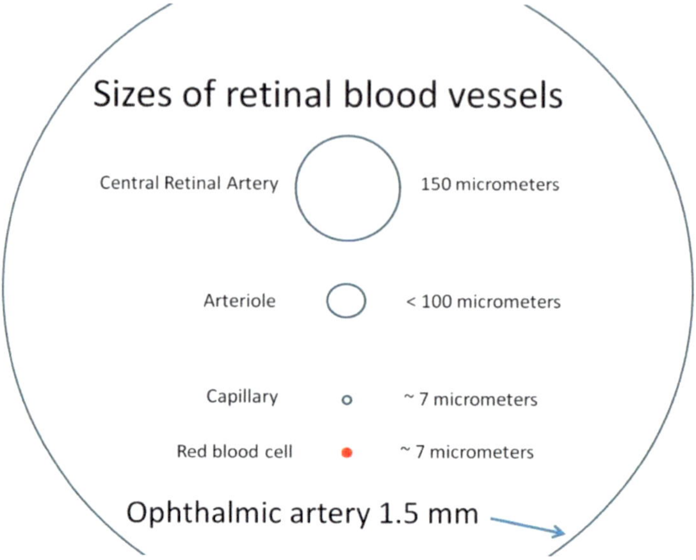


**Figure 131  Sizes of blood vessels**

At a diameter of 30 millimeters, the aorta is the largest artery in the body. The internal carotid artery is 5.8 millimeters in diameter. The ophthalmic artery, which supplies all of the blood to the eye, is 1.5 mm wide. The main artery entering the eye is the central retinal artery. At ~160 micrometers wide, it is only twice as wide as a human hair (around 80 micrometers). The retinal vessels carrying arterial blood range in size down to the capillaries, which are about the same size as a red blood cell (7 micrometers). The direct ophthalmoscope can resolve details which are around 25 micrometers in size: things smaller than that (such as capillaries or small aneurysms) cannot be seen.

The two major diseases affecting retinal blood vessels are hypertension and diabetes.

Hypertension has its major effects on arterioles, while diabetes has its major impact on capillaries. The walls of arterioles are quite muscular: a person with hypertension has chemicals in the blood which cause constriction of arterioles. When this is seen in the eye, the eye care professional will be alerted to a diagnosis of hypertension. The constriction may cause death of portions of the retina. High blood pressure may also cause bleeding (hemorrhage) from retinal vessels.

For diabetic people, the thickening of capillary walls interferes with nourishment of tissues and with normal body defences; for example, white blood cells may have a hard time entering tissues to defend against infection. The reduced blood supply may also prompt the growth of new blood vessels, which are weaker than the original ones; therefore, there may be leakage of fluid or even blood into the eye, which will disturb vision. In diabetic people, high blood sugar may cause swelling of the lens in the eye, causing the eye to become more myopic. When blood sugar returns to normal, this effect decreases. Once blood sugar levels are stabilized, it is possible to come up with an accurate prescription for eyeglasses.

The retinal capillary layers are supplied by branches of the central retinal artery. Close to the Optic Nerve Head, where the nerve fiber layer is thickest, there may be three or four layers of capillaries within the thickness of the retina. Away from the nerve head, there are fewer capillary layers, until you reach the foveal region, where there are no capillaries at all. Capillaries have walls which are one cell thick, and these walls have other cells (pericytes) wrapped around them to give some strength.

In diabetes, the capillary walls become thickened (which interferes with normal blood-borne defences), and the pericytes are gradually lost (allowing the walls to balloon outward, forming aneurysms). Aneurysms in diabetes may range in size from 7 micrometers to hundreds of micrometers. Considering the resolving power of the direct ophthalmoscope, aneurysms may be present but not visible. Aneurysms may become filled with platelets from the blood, which will make them disappear.

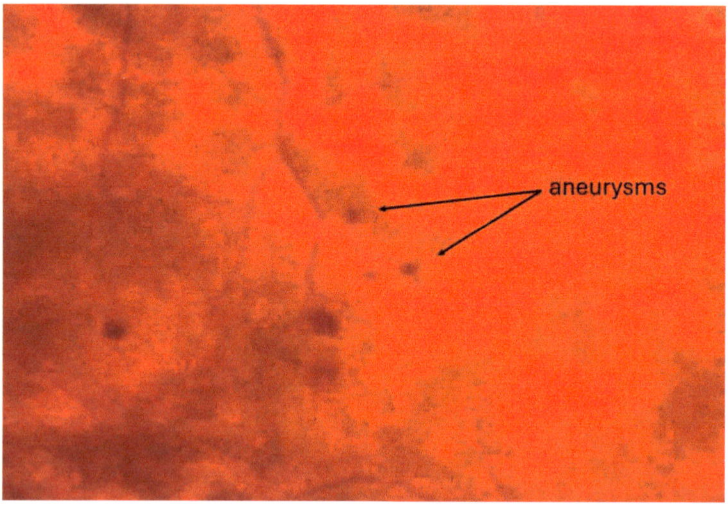


Figure 132 Aneurysms in diabetes

**Aneurysms in the retina of a person with long-standing (~10 years) diabetes**

The large arterioles (upper left of picture) are about 100 micrometers in diameter. Retinal arterioles are surrounded by a 150 micrometer-wide capillary-free zone, because the retina may be nourished directly by nutrients which diffuse directly across the wall of the arteriole. Farther from the arteriole, capillaries are present. The capillaries are about 6 micrometers across, which is below the usual resolving power of the direct ophthalmoscope, so they are not seen. These aneurysms (on capillaries) are at a distance from the adjacent arteriole. The 150 micrometer distance is about equal to the width of the central retinal artery trunk. Other red spots closer to arterioles are hemorrhages which have originated from damaged capillaries, but have the ability to move around within the retina. Individual hemorrhages may disappear because of phagocytic activity of the retinal microglial cells (the phagocytic, immunocompetent cells found throughout the central nervous system).

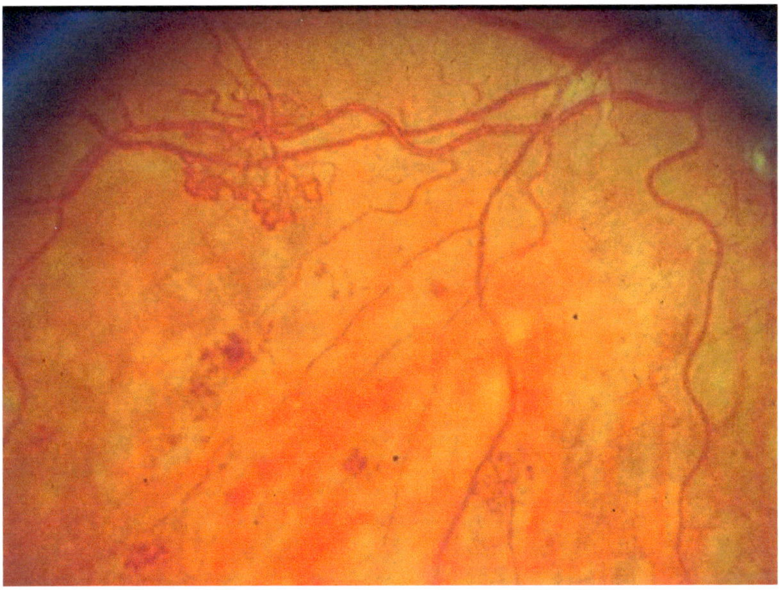

Figure 133 New blood vessel growth in diabetes

## New blood vessel formation in long-standing diabetes

When the original capillaries become thickened by diabetes, the tissues are starved of nourishment, which, after 10 years or so, is a stimulus to the body to make new blood vessels. At the top of this image, there is a net-like area of new blood vessel growth. While these new blood vessels will help to nourish the retina, they are not as strong as the original ones, and have a tendency to bleed. Some of the new blood vessels are within the retina, while some are on top, between the vitreous and the retina. Bleeding on top of the retina or into the vitreous is a serious problem. Not only does the blood obstruct vision, but it may clot and contract, pulling the retina off the retinal pigment epithelium.

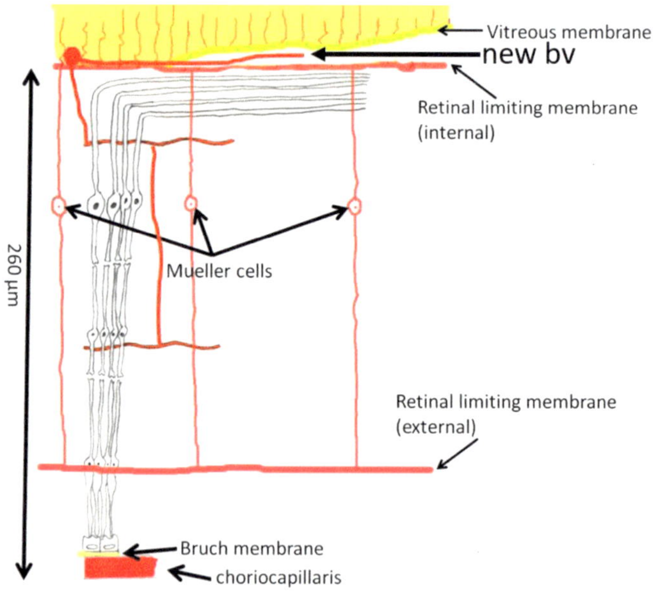


Figure 134 Growth of new blood vessels between internal limiting membrane and vitreous

To control growth of new blood vessels, a laser may be used to heat up and seal off the new blood vessels. Alternatively, agents which inhibit growth of new blood vessels may be injected into the vitreous. Both methods are currently in use.

# HYPERTENSION

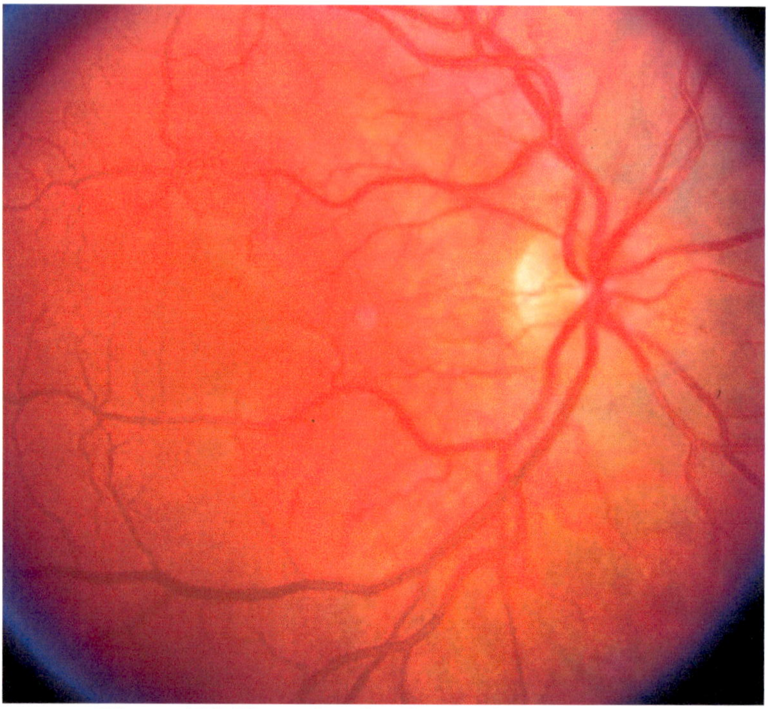

**Figure 135 Normal ratio of artery/vein diameters**

Here is a view of a normal nerve head and retinal blood vessels. The vessels which nourish the retina closer to the inside of the eye (the central retinal artery and central retinal vein) make their entrance and exit at the nerve head. At the nerve head, the central retinal artery branches into arterioles which run over the surface of the retina. They are redder than the veins and normally slightly smaller than the veins: a normal size ratio would be 3:4. Note how the upper arteriole criss-crosses the underlying vein. (By definition, an arterial blood vessel with a diameter under 100 micrometers is an arteriole.)

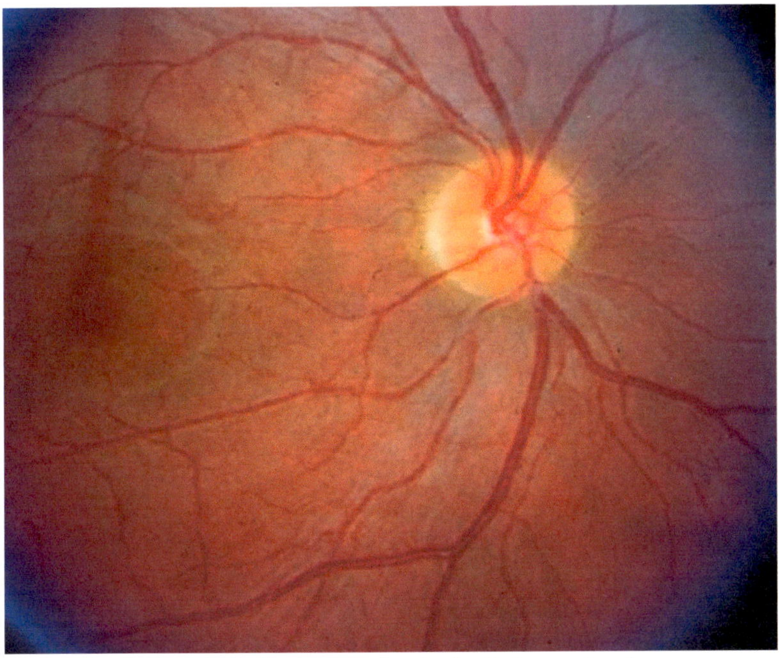

Figure 136 Constricted arteries in hypertension

In hypertension, the muscles of the arterioles contract, causing a narrowing of the blood vessel. This increases the resistance to blood flow, which must be compensated by increasing effort of the heart to pump blood through the tissues. This results in increased blood pressure throughout the body. Compare the diameters of the arterioles in this image with those of the preceding one. The arterioles in this picture are more like 1/3 or even 1/4 of the diameter of the veins. This person has hypertension.

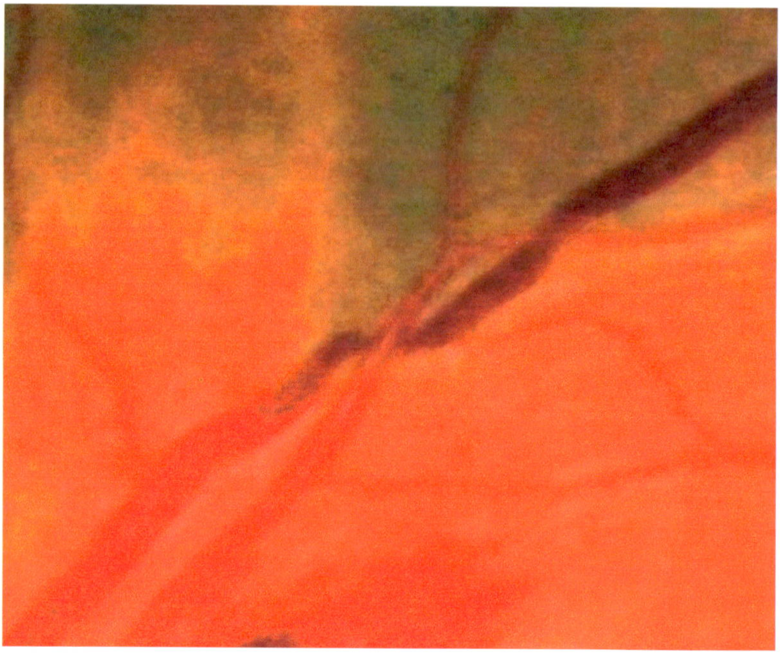

Figure 137 Compression of vein by overlying, hardened artery

Longstanding high blood pressure causes thickening of the walls of arteries and arterioles, with the result that they can compress veins they pass over. In this hypertensive person, the hardened arteriole is compressing the vein. Some vein compression may be seen here at both points where the artery passes on top of the vein. Hemorrhages are common in hypertension, and there is evidence of a hemorrhage at the bottom of this view.

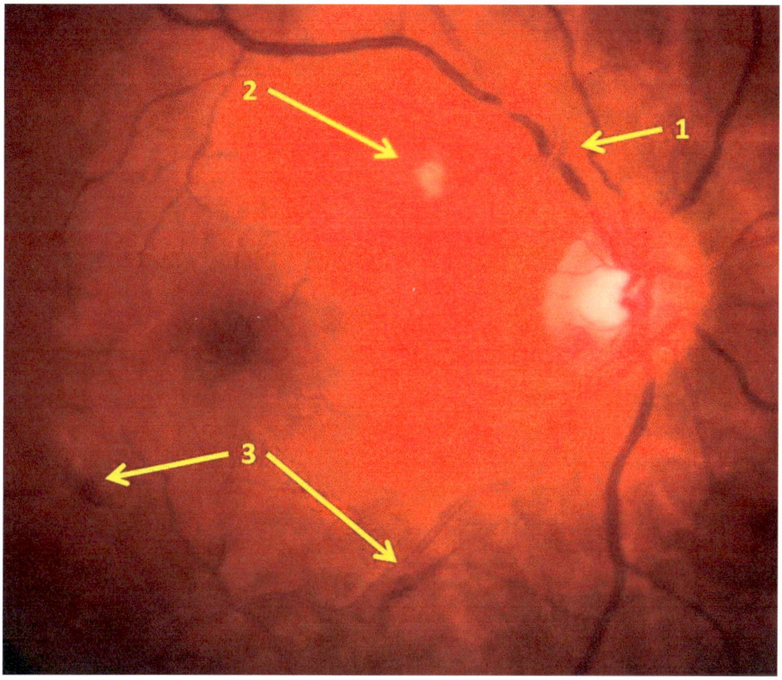


Figure 138 Retinal signs of hypertension

This person was indifferent to his health, and had been living with undetected hypertension for years. At the point marked '1', compression of the vein by the hardened arteriole is visible. At the points marked '3', there are hemorrhages within the retina. By the head of the arrow from '2', a small area of retinal nerve fiber layer has died, and the ganglion cells toward the left of the picture (say near where the start of the arrow appears) are still sending materials via orthograde axoplasmic flow toward the Optic Nerve Head, with the resultant appearance of a small white, fluffy cloud at the head of arrow 2, where the materials have accumulated upstream from the damaged axons. Over time, the microglial cells of the retina will remove this fluffy area.

# Chapter 8 AGING AND THE EYE

## DRY EYE

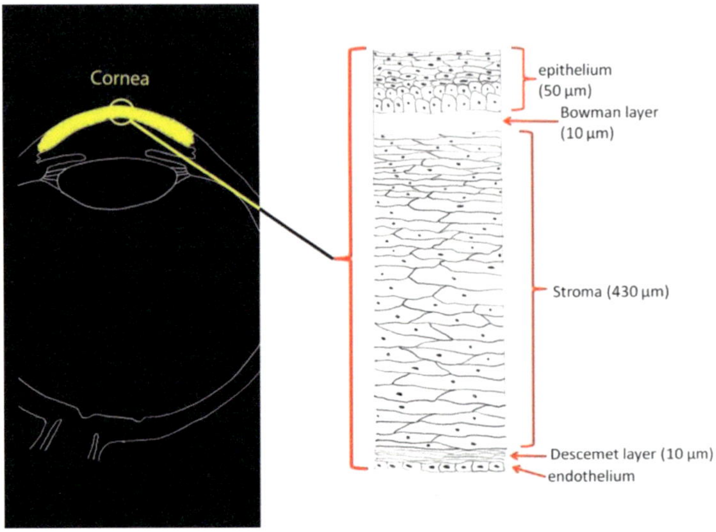


**Figure 139 Corneal detail**

Dry eye is a problem affecting the corneal epithelium and its overlying layers of mucus, tears and oil. The epithelium has the same structure as skin, with new cells forming just above the Bowman layer, and gradually flattening as they move to the surface, where they eventually fall off. Most of the corneal thickness is stroma. The tough, elastic Descemet layer lies at the bottom of the stroma. The hard-working endothelium is at the bottom of this diagram: its job is to pump water out of the whole cornea. The total corneal thickness is 500 micrometers, and the 50-micrometer thick corneal epithelium is very sensitive to any kind of injury: it has more nerve endings per square millimeter than any other part of the body. If it becomes dry, it's very uncomfortable. A healthy cornea also depends on the health of the sensory nerves which serve it.

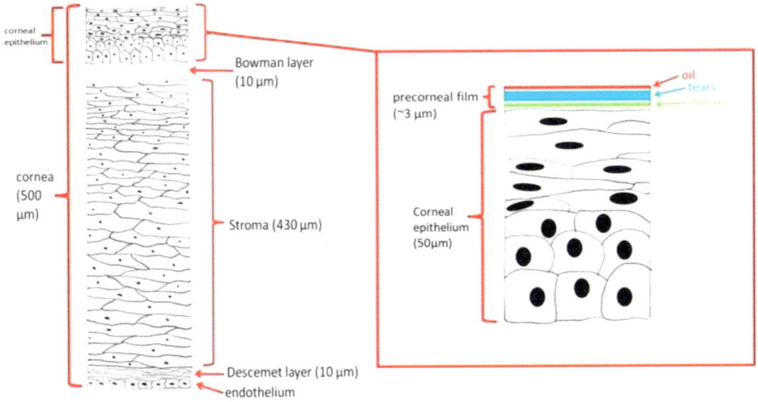


**Figure 140 Precorneal film**

Figure 140 shows more detail regarding the corneal epithelium and the precorneal film which lies on top. Dry eye is a problem involving the precorneal film. All three layers need to be present in the right proportion for the eye to be comfortable. The bottom layer of the precorneal film (green) is mucus, which fills in any gaps in the top layer of the epithelium. Each time you blink, you are polishing the front surface of the cornea. The middle layer (blue) is tears, which come from the lacrimal glands near the upper, outer corner of the eye. If there is a decrease in tear production (as in rheumatoid arthritis or lupus), the eye will be uncomfortable.

The top layer (red) is oil, which is produced by the Meibomian glands in the lids: its major function is to stop evaporation of the tear layer. If there is too little oil, the eye will feel dry, even though there are lots of tears for the middle layer. If there is too much oil, it may cause some blurriness of vision, and the oil itself in large quantities is acidic and can be quite irritating. If there is too little oil, the tears will evaporate too quickly.

Artificial tears can supplement the tear layer and also contain an agent which supplements the action of the oil layer. When you have dry eye, artificial tears should be used frequently throughout the day, not just when the eye becomes uncomfortable. For many people, decreased blinking due to long-term screen or tablet use is a cause of dry eye symptoms. Dry eye symptoms may also be caused by inflammation, in those cases, anti-inflammatory drops are needed. The use of lubricants containing vasoconstrictors is unwise because of a tendency for rebound eye redness.

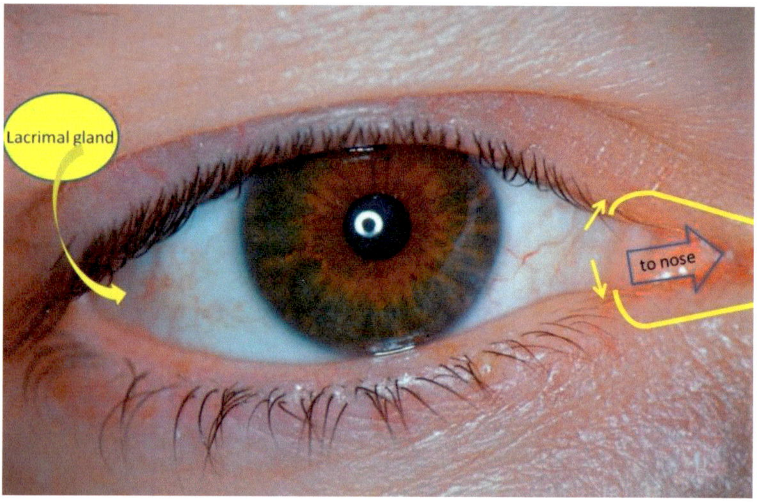


**Figure 141 normal flow of tears**

The lacrimal gland is in the orbit and eyelid near the outer corner of the eye. A normal dietary supply of vitamin A is necessary for the health of the lacrimal gland. Tears formed by the lacrimal gland are released onto the surface of the eye near the outer corner of the eye. They flow over the surface of the eye and then enter the tear drainage system close to the nose.

The entry points to the drainage system (near the heads of the straight yellow arrows) are called the puncta. Tears pass through the upper and lower punctum to enter a fine tube which conducts them toward the nose. The open blue arrow in this diagram lies over the inner canthus of the eye, and the curved yellow arrow also indicates the outer canthus of the eye. Severe vitamin A deficiency can cause dryness (xerosis) and potential vision loss. Worldwide, vitamin A deficiency is a significant cause of vision loss.

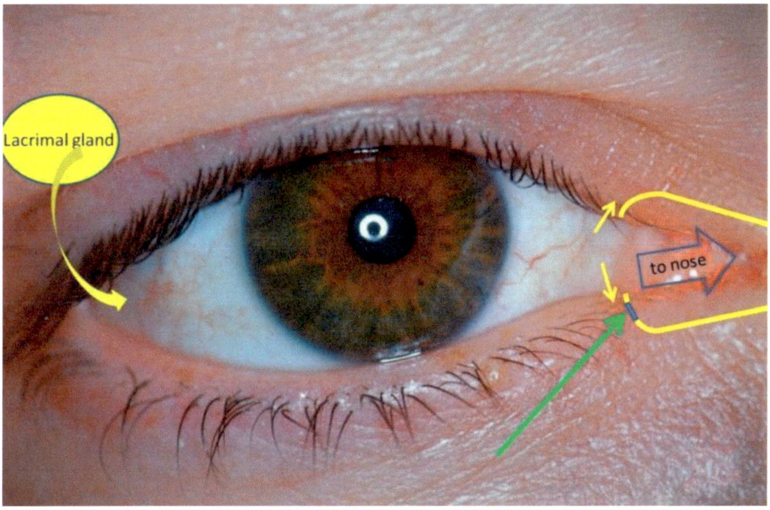


**Figure 142 Blocking punctum to increase tear availability.**

If dry eye is caused by decreased production of tears by the lacrimal gland, it may be possible to increase the available tear volume by decreasing the outflow of tears into the nose. This can be done on a trial basis using a plug made of dissolvable collagen (a punctal plug).
The plug is inserted through the punctum (the entry point of the drainage system) and sits in the position shown by the green arrow. If this temporary plug gives relief from dry eye symptoms, then a permanent plug, made of silicone,

may be used. Punctal plugs may be placed through the upper or lower punctum, or both puncta if necessary.

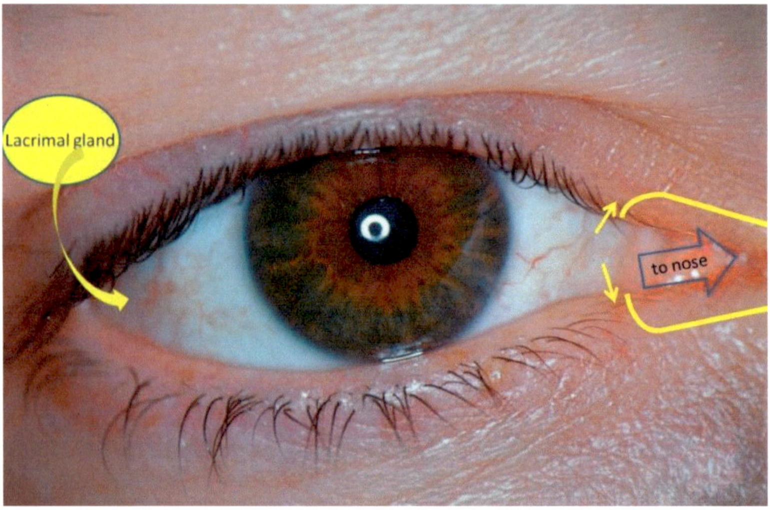


Figure 143 Normal tear flow

## TEARY EYE

Under normal conditions, there are enough tears to contribute to the tear layer of the precorneal film and maintain the normal wetting of the eye, and the drainage system is working well enough to remove the tears into the nose. If there is increased tear production (for example due to emotional stimuli or preparing onions), then the tears may overflow and run down the eyelid. It is good practice for anyone with a teary eye to dry the eye always by moving a tissue upward. Frequent downward pulling of the eyelid, particularly in an older person, may encourage the eyelid to droop downward, away from the eyeball. If this droop is severe enough, plastic surgery may be needed to tighten the lower lid. (Sometimes the skin of the upper lid may start to hang over the lid margin, and this may also be corrected with further plastic surgery.)

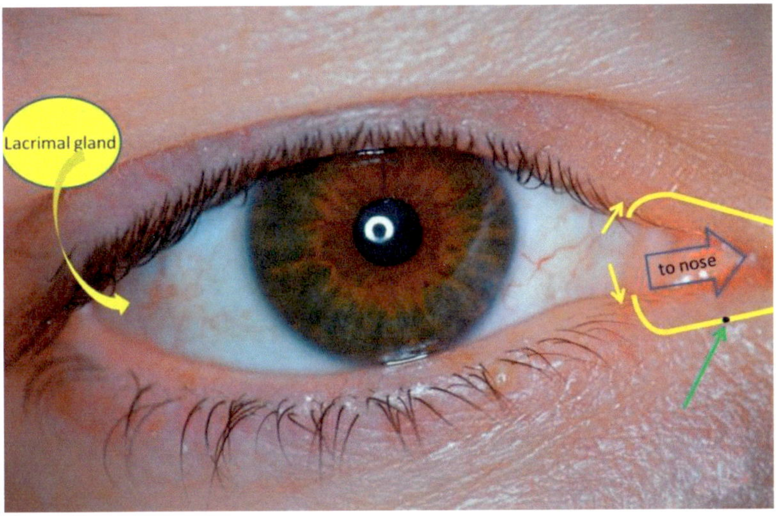


Figure 144 Blocked nasolacrimal duct

If there is tearing due to blockage of the drainage system (shown by green arrow), the offending material may be flushed through into the nose. This is done by inserting a very fine tube through the punctum and introducing saline into the drainage system. Usually, the material causing the blockage is easily pushed out of the system, into the nose.

## VITREOUS DETACHMENT

There are connections between the vitreous humor and the retinal internal limiting membrane. The Mueller cells of the retina are structural cells which help to hold the retina together. They run through the full thickness of the retina and produce the two limiting membranes shown here. The internal and external segments of the photoreceptors pass through the external limiting membrane. The vitreous is anchored to the internal limiting membrane by means of fine collagen strands which are secreted by the Mueller cells. When the vitreous detaches from the internal limiting membrane (a normal, age-related event), these fine collagen strands will break. As they break, there will be traction on the retina, which may result in perception of flashing lights.

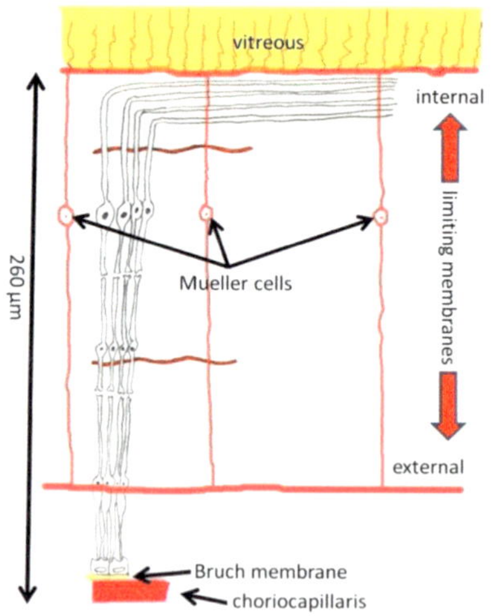


**Figure 145 Normal vitreous attachments**

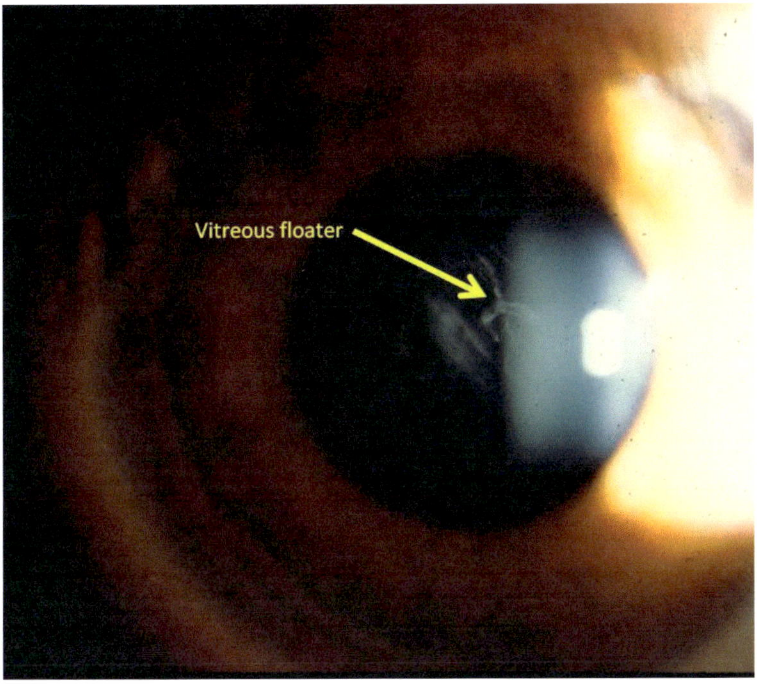


Figure 146 Vitreous floaters

Using the slit lamp to focus in the plane behind the crystalline lens, it is possible to see some fine membranes floating in the vitreous just behind the lens. The light from the slit lamp is entering the eye from the right of this picture, and the iris and lens are both out of focus because focus is on the floaters.

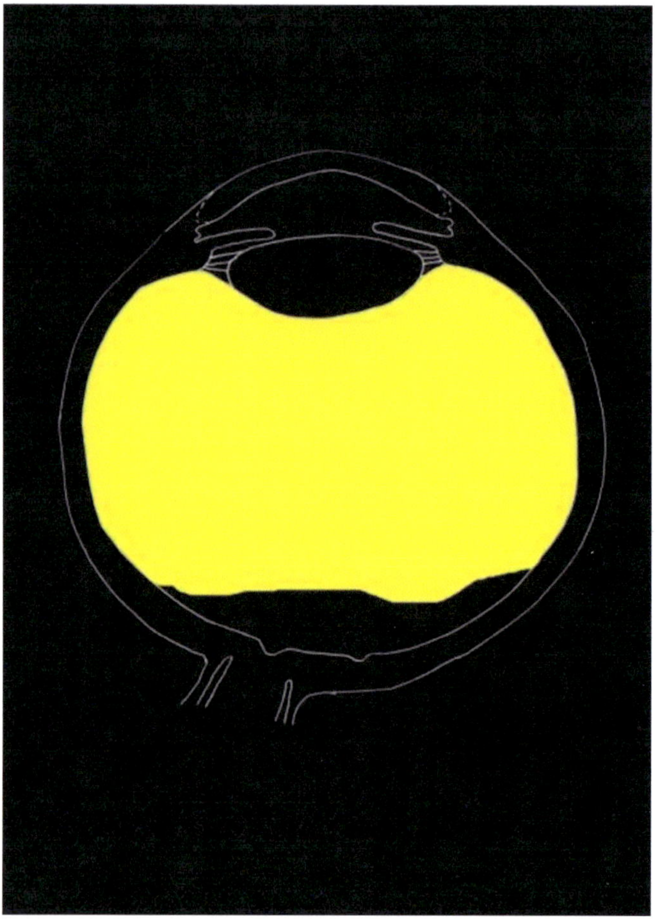

Figure 147 Posterior vitreous detachment

The vitreous humor consists of collagen (protein), hyaluronic acid, and water. With age, the collagen tends to clump together and release the water, much as a squeezed sponge releases the water it contains. As a result, the more solid part of the vitreous tends to move toward the front of the eye (the strongest attachment of the vitreous is by the ciliary body at the front of the eye), while the water pools in the space between the vitreous and the retina at the back of the eye. The normal vitreous contains a number of pieces left over from the embryonic development of the eye (bits of intravitreal blood vessels, for example). As the vitreous becomes more liquid, these pieces are allowed to float free and cast shadows on the retina.

When the vitreous detaches, the fine collagen strands of the vitreous break away from their attachment to the internal limiting membrane, which causes traction on the retina, and causes the patient to experience flashing lights (photopsia). In most cases, posterior vitreous detachment is a normal age-related change; however, it is always necessary to rule out retinal detachment when there are symptoms of flashing lights. The same caution must be taken when there is appearance of many new floaters.

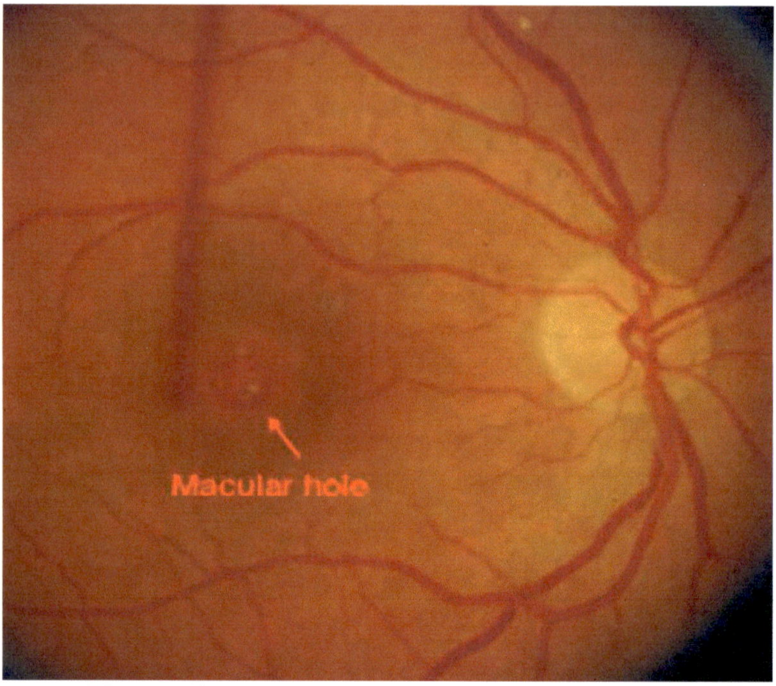


Figure 148 Macular hole due to vitreous detachment

If there is a stronger than usual ring attachment between the vitreous and the macular area, vitreous detachment may pull a hole in the retina, causing a reduction in visual acuity.

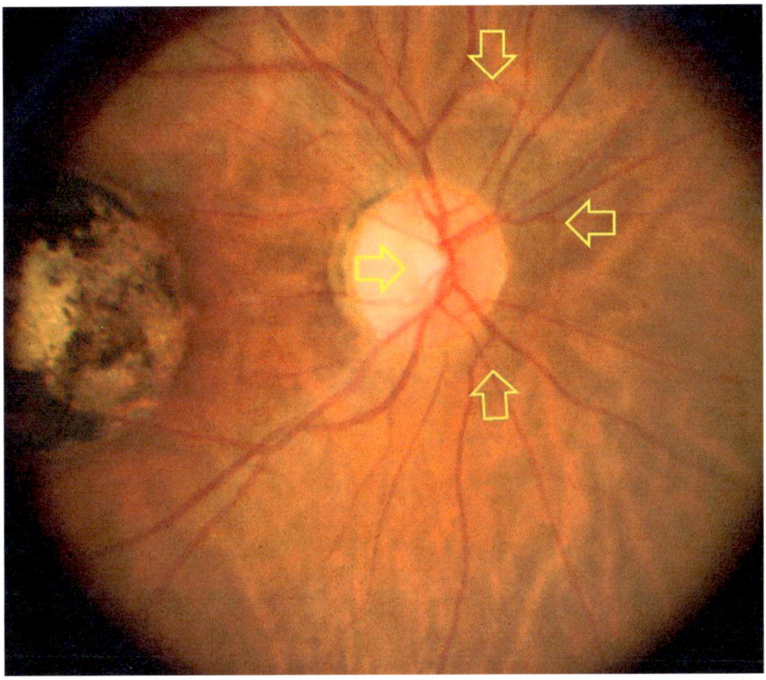

Figure 149 Ring attachment came off nerve head because of inflammation

This patient lost the central vision of the right eye ten years previously, due to a retinal inflammation (Retinochoroiditis) caused by the protozoan, *Toxoplasma gondii* (the disease is called toxoplasmosis). The area of black scar tissue on the left (due to retinal pigment epithelial reaction to the infection) is centered on the fovea. The violent inflammation of the retina and vitreous caused a posterior vitreous detachment.

The yellow arrows point out a translucent, ellipse-shaped structure floating in the vitreous. Originally, this was the circular attachment of the vitreous to the Optic Nerve Head: over time it has shifted toward the front of the eye and become distorted.

People who have normal, age-related posterior vitreous detachments are often initially aware of a circular shadow floating in their vision, and this is its origin. With time, ring floater(s) may become less noticeable, as they shift toward the front of the eye and cast a fainter shadow.

## PRESBYOPIA (this word means literally, 'old eye'.)

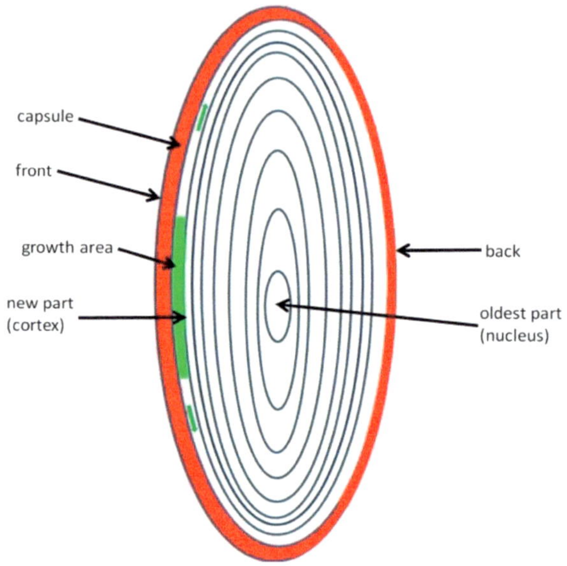


**Figure 150 Lens structure**

On the left side of Figure 39, you can see the optic cup having an interesting impact on the overlying surface ectoderm. It first thickens to form the lens placode, which then infolds (much as the neuroectoderm does), later separating from the surface ectoderm to form the hollow lens vesicle about 30 days after conception. Growth of lens fibers obliterates the empty center of the vesicle, producing a solid lens. It is the influence of the optic cup which induces these changes in the surface ectoderm. Under normal conditions, the lens sits there at the front of the eye for about 40 years, doing its job perfectly.

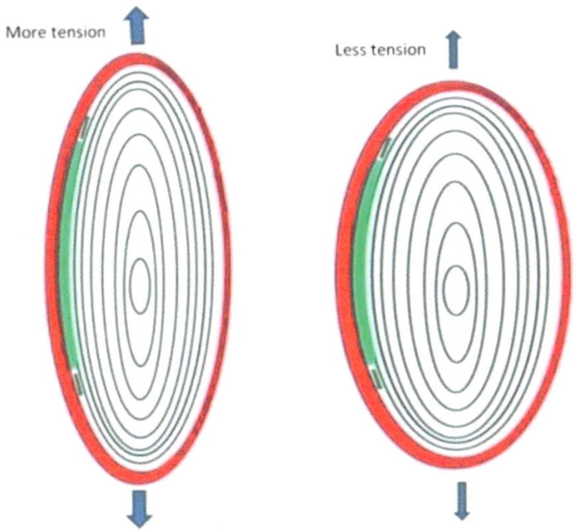


Figure 151 Lens changes shape during accommodation

However, the lens grows as a tree grows: new layers are added from the outside (cortex). The growth area is shown in green. New fibers follow the path of the green arrows, almost completely surrounding the older layers. The older layers gradually move toward the centre (nucleus). As they move inward, the lens fibers gradually lose their nuclei.

Injury to the eye (for example blunt trauma or chemical injury) may cause the outermost layer of the lens to become opaque to some extent. Later, normal layers of fibers are laid down over the opaque layer. Because of this tree-like growth, it is possible to recognize the age at which the opacities were caused, just as tree experts can recognize good years and bad years in a tree's growth. (The lens at age 10 is 3 mm thick, and 6 mm at age 80.) The young lens is pliable and can be squeezed into a rounder shape by the elastic capsule, which is thicker at the front than the back.

Figure 151 shows how we change our focus from a distant object to a near one. The lens is suspended from the circular ciliary muscle of the ciliary body. When that muscle is relaxed (left side of diagram), there is increased tension on the lens capsule, pulling the lens into a flatter shape of lower focal power. When the ciliary muscle contracts, the tension on the lens capsule is decreased (right side of diagram), allowing the elastic capsule to deform the lens into a rounder shape, with higher focal power.

The lens gets thicker and stiffer with age: around age 40, the lens can't change its shape enough for you to see at arm's length (unless you happen to be short-sighted). The clarity of the lens depends on the orderliness of its layers: in time, the layers start to scatter some light. With age, the lens starts to filter out the short wavelengths, so blues appear less intense. The lens you were born with is very good at filtering short wavelengths, particularly ultraviolet (UV).

After cataract surgery, this protection from UV is reduced, and you should wear sunglasses to protect the retina, particularly the macula, from harmful UV exposure.

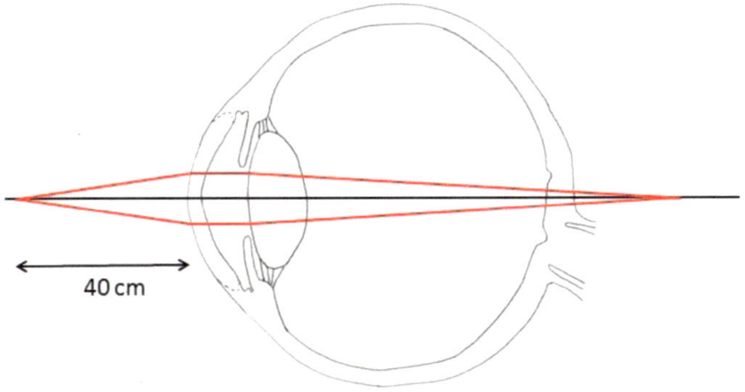


Figure 152 Young presbyope

Figure 152 shows a ~45-year-old eye which can see clearly at distance with no lenses. This person has lost some ability to change lens power (accommodation) because of thickening and stiffness of the lens inside the eye. When this person looks at an object at 40 cm (16 inches or arm's length), the image falls behind the retina and is blurry.

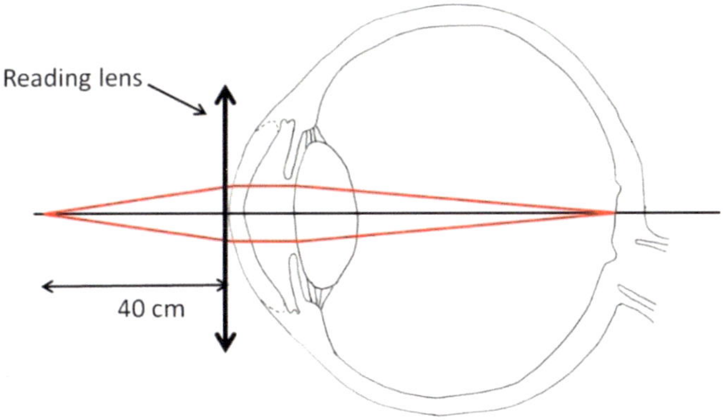


Figure 153 Older presbyope

A relatively low power reading lens (around +1.00 D for example) will clear up near vision.

As the lens becomes increasingly stiff, the reading lens power needed will gradually increase until around age 60, when nearly all accommodation is lost.
When a person puts on a reading lens, the object at 40 cm is seen clearly: the lens is increasing the eye's focal power and making up for lost accommodation. The focal power of this reading lens for a 60 year old is 1/0.4 = +2.50 diopters. If this same person wished to see clearly at 20 cm, they would need a lens of power 1/0.2 = +5.00 diopters. If a person were myopic and required a -2.50 diopter lens to see in the distance, and wanted to see things at 40 cm from their eyes, all they would have to do is take off their glasses.

Until reading lenses were discovered, many people just gave up reading, or had someone read things to them. Somewhere in the 13$^{th}$ century, people began to use glasses for reading. The use of lenses to help clear up distance vision did not occur until about 2 centuries later. The last of optical eye problems to be conquered was astigmatism, in the 19$^{th}$ century.

## CATARACT

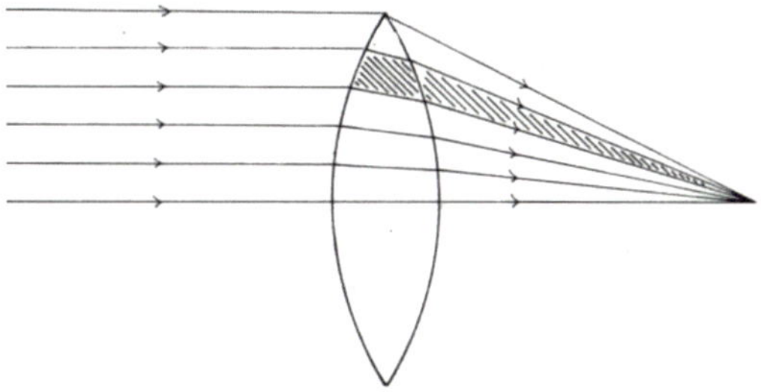

Figure 154 Lens opacity doesn't block whole image

The term 'cataract' is best used to describe the situation where there are so many opacities in the lens that there is an impact on a person's daily life. Many people with lens opacities never reach the point where they need surgery.

If this lens has a cloudy area in it, the rest of the lens is capable of producing a complete image: each part of the lens produces a complete image. The effect of the blocking of some of the light will be that the brightness of the image will be slightly reduced.

## THE SLIT LAMP

Here is how the slit lamp works. In the top sketch, you can see a horizontal section of the eye, viewed from above. The slit lamp has an ingenious light source which is being used to aim a narrow vertical sheet of light into the eye. The direction of this beam of illumination (see arrow marked 'ILLUM') can be changed, depending on what you want to see. In this drawing, the vertical sheet of light has been turned to the left. (If the slit beam were directed straight at the eye, the structures in the lower diagram would all be on top each other, and no thicknesses could be seen!) The slit lamp also includes a fine binocular microscope which can be used to examine structures of the eye at many different magnifications.

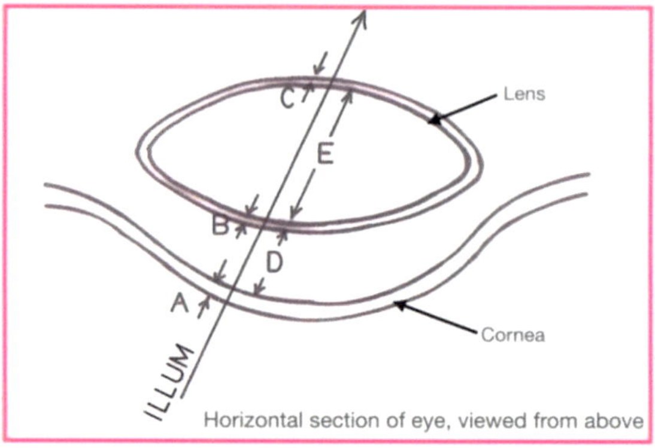


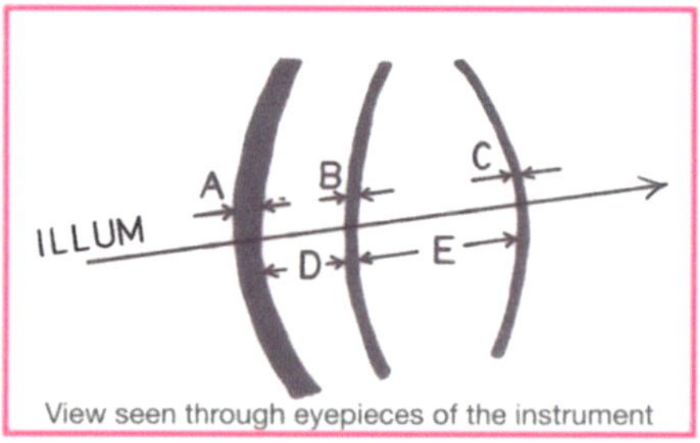


Figure 155 Looking at front of eye with Slit Lamp

In the bottom view is a sketch of what the examiner sees through the eyepieces of the microscope. It is as though you are seeing a 'slice' of the structures of the eye.

The thicknesses of the eye structures are shown in both drawings:
A is the thickness of the cornea
B is the thickness of the front capsule of the lens
C is the thickness of the rear capsule of the lens
D is the depth of the anterior chamber
E is the thickness of the lens

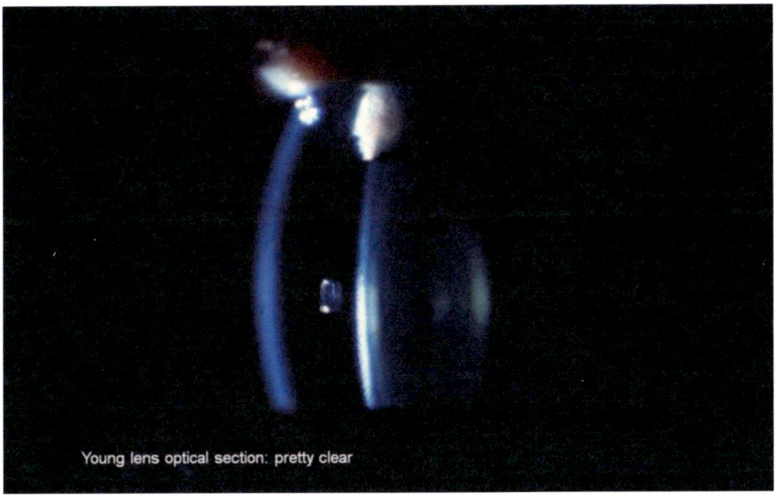


Figure 156 Optical Section of lens

The clarity of the lens depends on an orderly arrangement of its fibers. If this arrangement if disturbed, then scattering of light happens. If there is enough scattering, there will be an opacity in the lens.

## POSTERIOR SUBCAPSULAR CATARACT

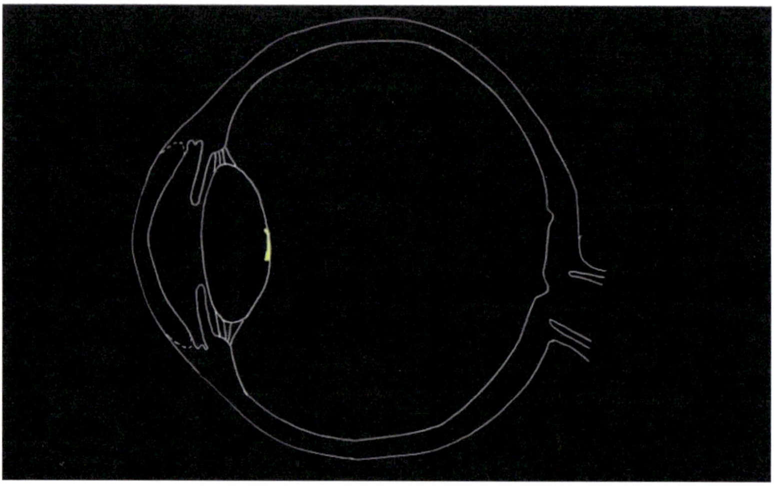

**Figure 157 Sketch of posterior subcapsular cataract**

The posterior lens capsule is relatively thin, and a posterior subcapsular cataract may develop due to age, trauma, steroid use, alcohol abuse, and inflammation. These situations appear to interfere with the orderly laying down of developing lens fibers as they approach the posterior pole of the lens.

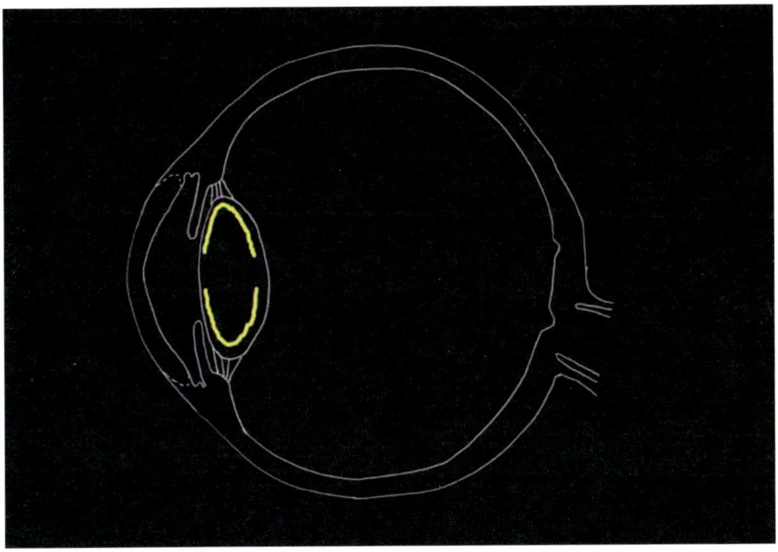

**Figure 158 Sketch of cortical cataract**

## CORTICAL CATARACT

Some of the outer layers of lens are not lining up with others, so some scattering of light happens. When examined with the slit lamp, these scattering layers may appear like spokes moving from the edge of the lens toward the center of the pupil.

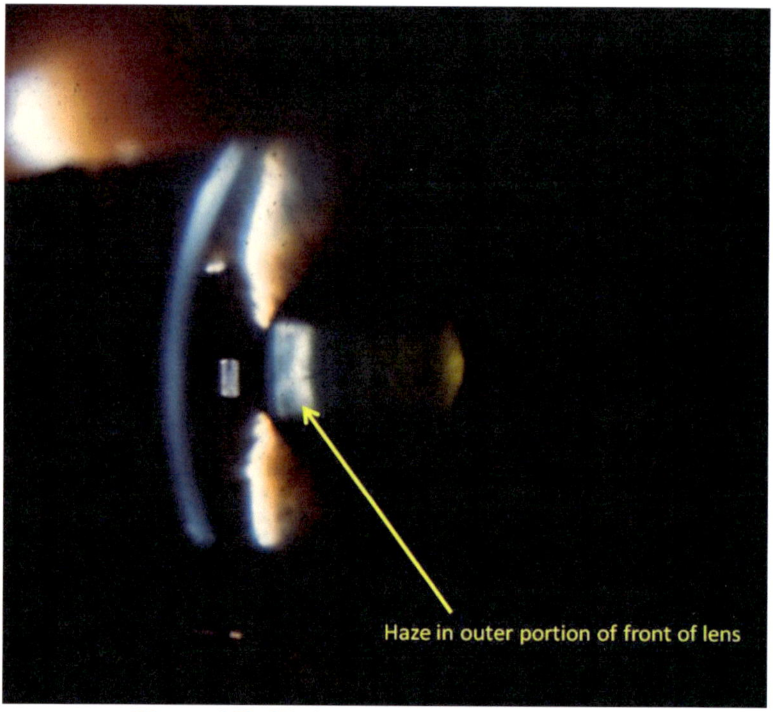


**Figure 159 Clinical view of cortical cataract**

Here is a view of a cataract which involves the cortex (outer portion) of the lens. The slit lamp is focused on the cortex at the front of the lens. Irregular layers of lens fibres in the cortex are scattering some light, while most of the nucleus is clear. In spite of the opacity, this person still had very good vision.

## NUCLEAR CATARACT

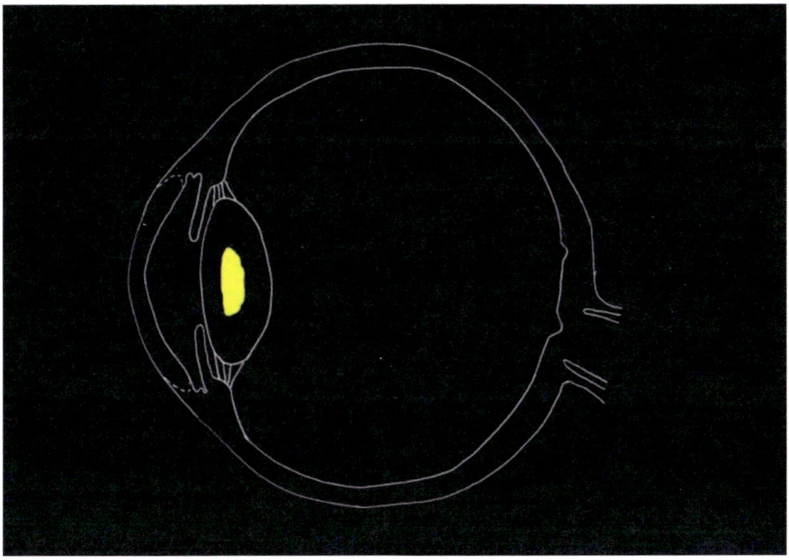

Figure 160 Sketch of nuclear cataract

Nuclear cataracts are less common than cortical cataracts, and tend to develop more quickly than cortical cataract. A person with nuclear cataract may go from having good vision to requiring cataract surgery in a year, while a person with cortical cataract may never reach the point where cataract surgery is required at all. Nuclear cataract has a greater impact on vision, as a larger percentage of the light reaching the retina has to pass through the center of the lens.

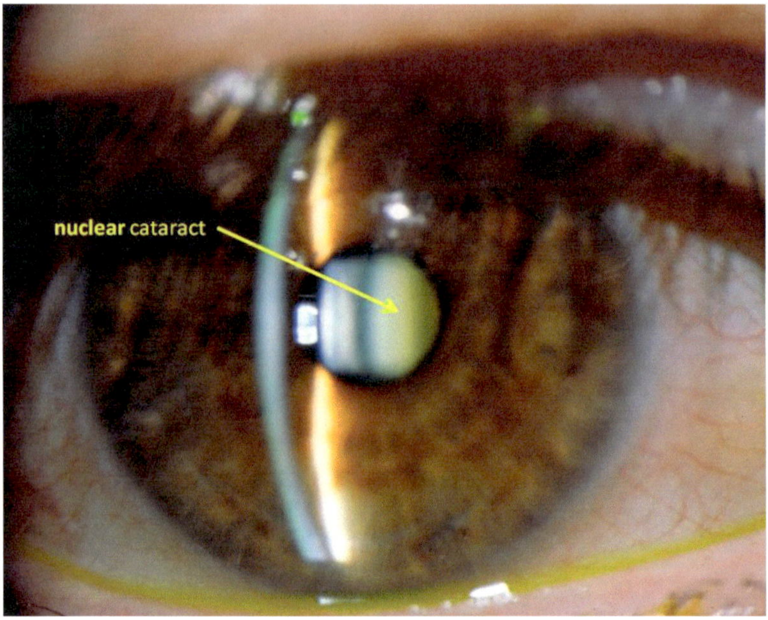


Figure 161 Clinical view of nuclear cataract

Here is a clinical view of a nuclear cataract. The center of the lens is looking rather brown. The main area of opacity in this lens is centered at the core (nucleus) of the lens. When a nuclear cataract is developing, there may be some swelling of the lens, which increases its focal power and makes the patient more near-sighted (or less far-sighted).

## CATARACT SURGERY

When the light scattering is seriously hampering vision, surgery is needed. The lens capsule is opened and the hazy lens removed. The lost power of the original crystalline lens is replaced with an intraocular lens, which is placed inside the original lens capsule.

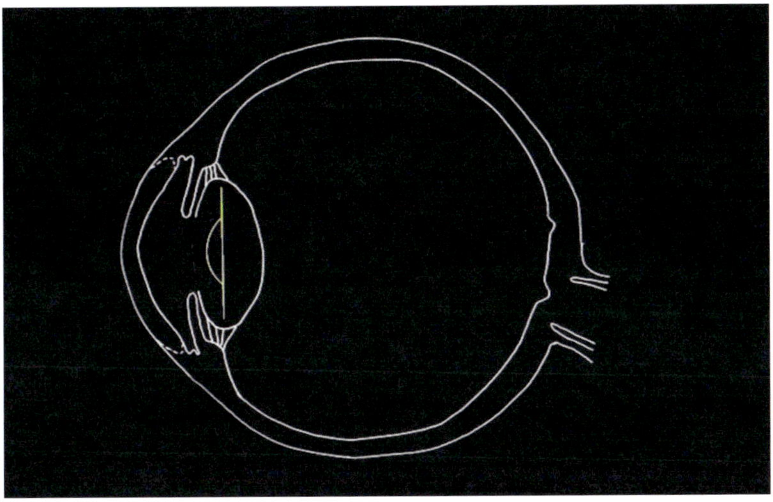

Figure 162 Placement of intraocular lens

## LASER CAPSULOTOMY

Cataract surgery leaves most of the capsule of the lens in place, with the intraocular lens placed inside the capsule. Approximately one in four patients who have cataract surgery experience some clouding of vision in the years following surgery, and this can be caused by a haziness of the capsule behind the intraocular lens. The haze arises because some of the lens material persists and starts growing again.

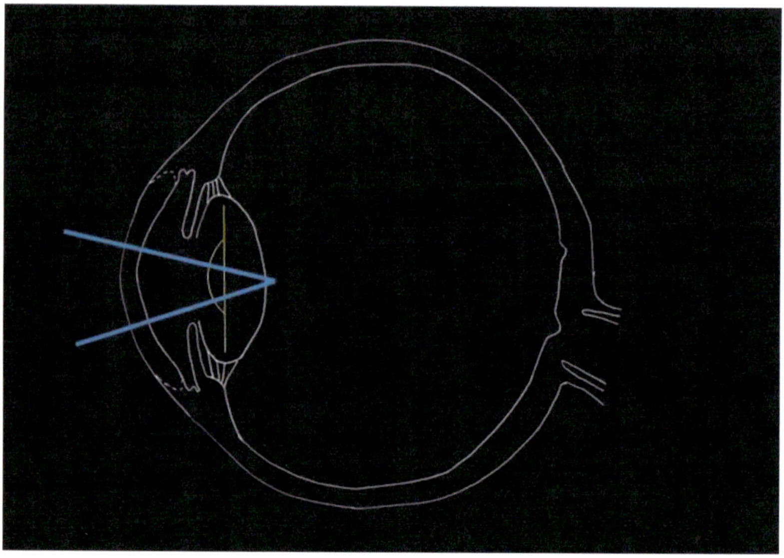

Figure 163 YAG laser focuses on rear lens capsule

If this is the cause of decreased vision, YAG laser treatment may be used to make a hole in the lens capsule behind the intraocular lens.

The type of laser used for closing new retinal blood vessels in cases of diabetes (an Argon laser) causes heat. The type of laser used to make a hole in the posterior capsule (a YAG laser or cold laser) causes a mechanical impact on the capsule.

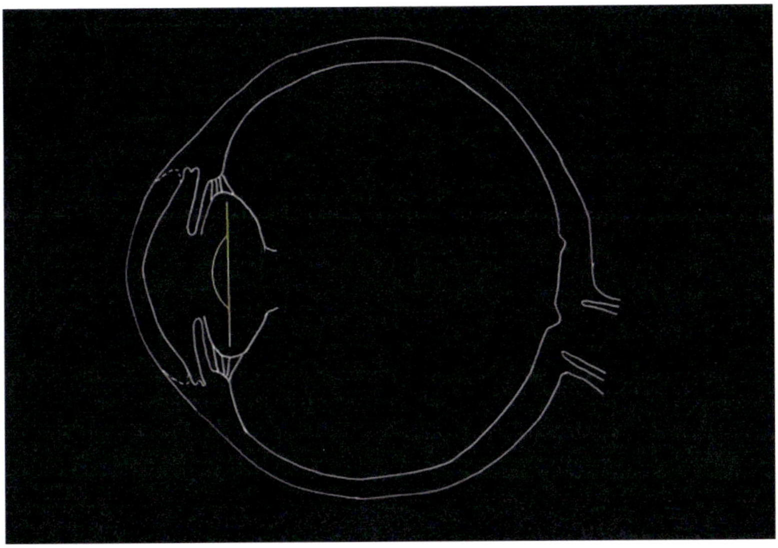

Figure 164 Opening in lens capsule improves vision

Following YAG laser treatment of hazy lens capsule (laser capsulotomy), an opening in the capsule allows clear vision through the intraocular lens.

## GLAUCOMA

This is a problem with its origin at the front of the eye and its effects at the back of the eye.

In the eye, fluid (called aqueous humor) is produced by highly vascular areas of the ciliary body (ciliary processes). This fluid travels as shown by red arrows in Figure 165 and drains into the venous system at the angle of the anterior chamber. If there is obstruction in the drainage system, the intraocular pressure rises and can damage the optic nerve: this is glaucoma. Damage to retinal ganglion cells and their axons may arise because of decreased blood supply or because of mechanical damage to the cells and their supporting astrocytes. The gradual vision loss in glaucoma may take years, and may not be noticed by the patient. In the majority of cases, the gradually increasing pressure in the eye causes no symptoms. Fortunately, there are drugs which can either decrease aqueous production or facilitate its drainage.

While most body tissues have a mechanical pressure of around 8 millimeters of mercury, the eye is unusual in having a pressure which normally ranges between 10 to 20 millimeters of mercury (around 15 mmHg on average). Intraocular pressure varies with the time of day (a diurnal change): it tends to be higher in the morning and lower in the afternoon. Blood pressure (BP) also shows a circadian rhythm, tending to be lower at night and higher during the day. In glaucoma, the intraocular pressure usually builds slowly over the space of several years. Because there are so many axons in the optic nerve, the effects of glaucoma are very slow in manifesting themselves. The effects of circadian rhythms (IOP and BP) may influence a diagnosis of glaucoma. Frequent checks of the visual field and measurements of retinal thickness are necessary before a diagnosis can be reached. Once a diagnosis of glaucoma

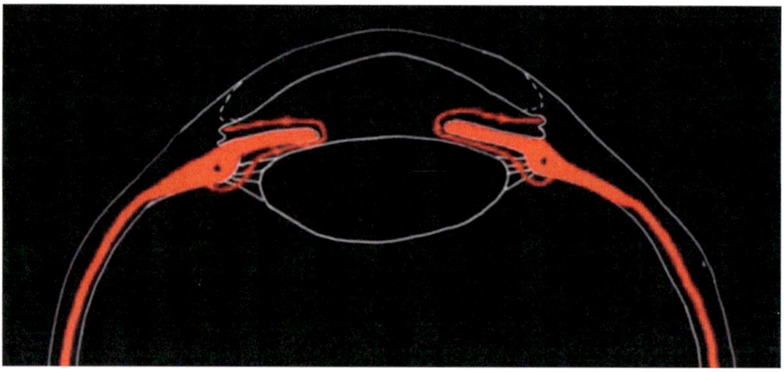

**Figure 165 Circulation of aqueous humor**

has been established, management involves lowering IOP by either decreasing production of aqueous or by increasing drainage of aqueous, and keeping watch on changes in the visual field and retinal thickness.

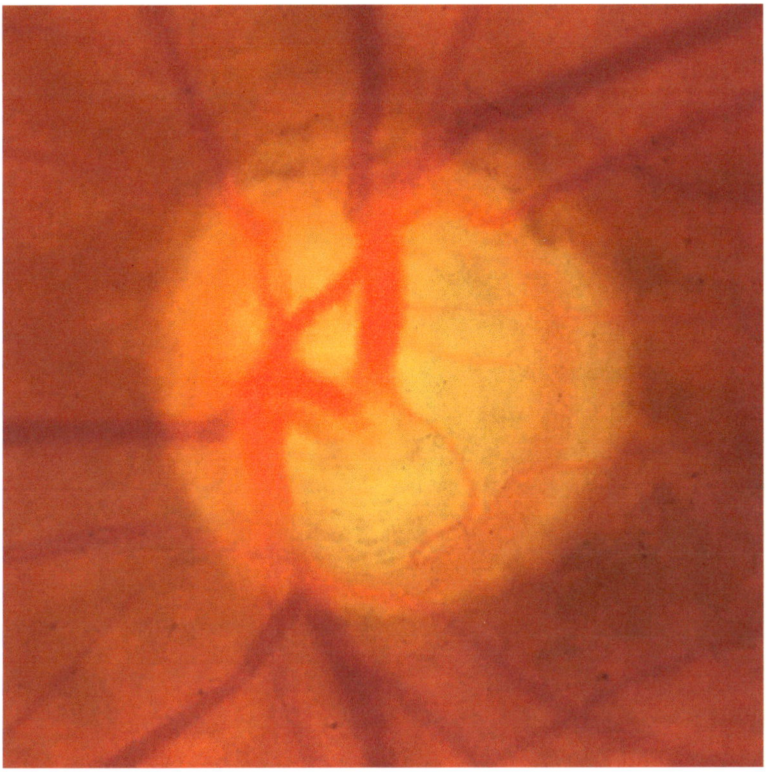

**Figure 166 Enlarged cupping due to axon loss in glaucoma**

Here is the Optic Nerve Head of a patient with established glaucoma in the left eye: note the large extent of lamina cribrosa visible at the bottom of the large cupping. The increased width and depth of the cupping is caused by loss of Ganglion Cell Axons, particularly at the lower edge of the nerve head. The axons lost from this area (the inferior part of the nerve head) are those which serve the upper (superior) part of the visual field, hence the constriction of the field in that area. The agreement of the physical appearance of the nerve head and the visual field supports the diagnosis of glaucoma.

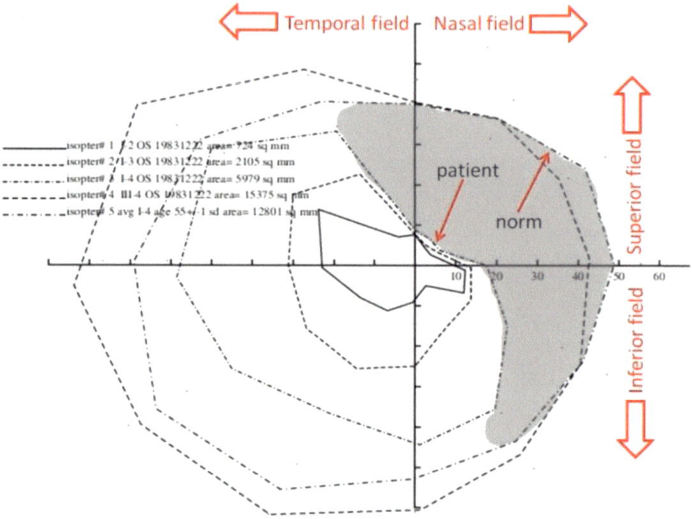


Goldmann Visual Field/file#

**Figure 167 Visual field loss in glaucoma**

Here is the visual field for the person shown in the previous image. The LEFT eye has been damaged by glaucoma. The inner three patterns show a considerable depression. As you move from the innermost pattern outward, the brightness of the test target is increased by 0.5 log unit, and there is little expansion of the second and third field tests. The narrow red arrows compare the patient's result (marked 'patient') with the average for his age group (marked 'norm'). If a very large, intense target (10 times brighter and 16 times larger than the first) is used, this patient's fourth visual field test result expands to a more normal shape. The gray area shows the extent of the lost visual field.

# MACULAR DEGENERATION

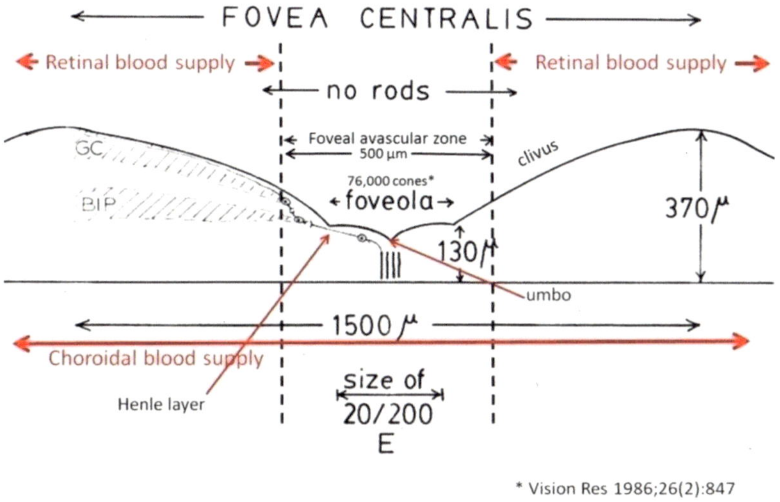


Figure 168 Dual blood supplies to retina except for fovea

Most of the retina has a dual blood supply, being sandwiched between the retinal and choroidal circulation. The foveal avascular zone (FAZ) has no capillaries from the retinal circulation, and is more vulnerable to the effects of decreased blood supply from the choroid. (The FAZ becomes widened in cases of diabetic retinopathy. There is a further suggestion that the FAZ may be widened in cases of glaucoma.) The FAZ occupies the central 1.7 degrees out of the whole visual field of at least 130 degrees for one eye (or 160 degrees for both eyes together). The rest of the retina, with its dual blood supply, is not threatened by macular degeneration. With suitable magnification, the peripheral retina can take over many of the functions of the macula if it is damaged.

Macular degeneration is usually 'dry' or 'wet'.

The dry variant (dry age-related macular degeneration) is the more common form, progresses slowly, and may take years to cause significant problems. Vitamin and lutein supplements may slow the development of macular degeneration (Evans JR, Lawrenson JG. Antioxidant vitamin and mineral supplements for slowing the progression of age-related macular degeneration. Cochrane Database of Systematic Reviews 2023, Issue 9. Art. No.: CD000254. DOI: 10.1002/14651858.CD000254.pub5. Accessed 13 January 2025.)
The wet variant (wet age-related macular degeneration), on the other hand, can cause rapid changes in vision and requires urgent treatment, usually aimed at blocking growth of new blood vessels.

**Figure 169 Congenital drusen**

A good approach to the problem of macular degeneration is to make lifestyle changes:

- routine wearing of sunglasses
- avoidance of
  - smoking,
  - sedentary lifestyle
  - highly-processed foods.

Figure 169 shows a right eye with numerous small, yellowish spots on the retina. These drusen-like spots were present at birth and have not changed over a period of many years. (Such spots may be present in a number of congenital conditions related to abnormal RPE function.) Drusen may also appear in adult life and may indicate decreased blood supply from the choriocapillaris. The following features of drusen have a better prognosis:

- smaller size
- smaller number
- farther from the foveal center
- more distinct outline

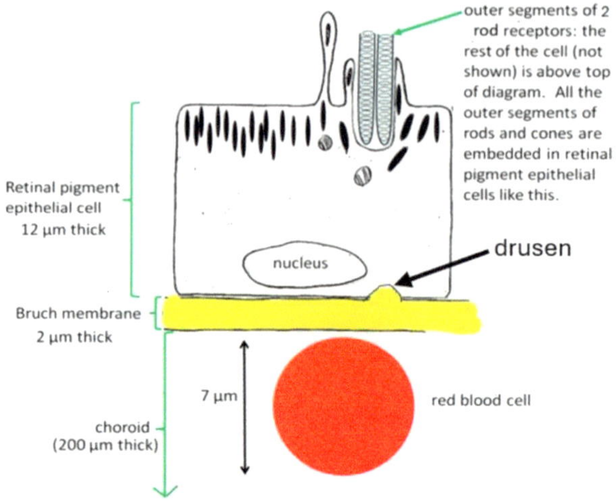


Figure 170 Sketch of drusen

Figure 170 is a sketch of a single drusen. It is caused by a thickening of Bruch membrane, which causes the overlying retinal pigment epithelial cell to be thinned. The higher the drusen, the larger the area of decreased retinal pigmentation.

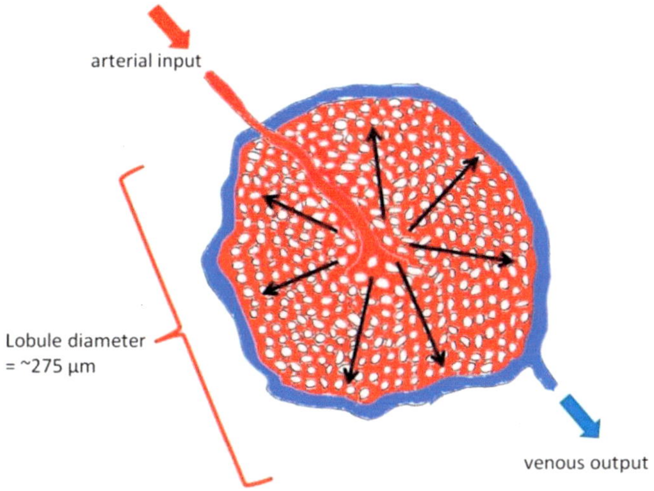


Figure 171 Lobule of choriocapillaris, Detail

Here is a sketch of a small portion of the choriocapillaris directly beneath the foveal center. The arterial blood is distributed to the fine capillaries of the choriocapillaris in a lobular pattern. It is delivered to the center of the lobule and then drains outward to the periphery. The average diameter of these lobules is 275 micrometers. If there is a reduced blood supply to the choriocapillaris, the flow to one lobule may be reduced; however, adjacent lobules may be able to take up the slack. Often visual function is still good, despite the ophthalmoscopic appearance of the macular area.

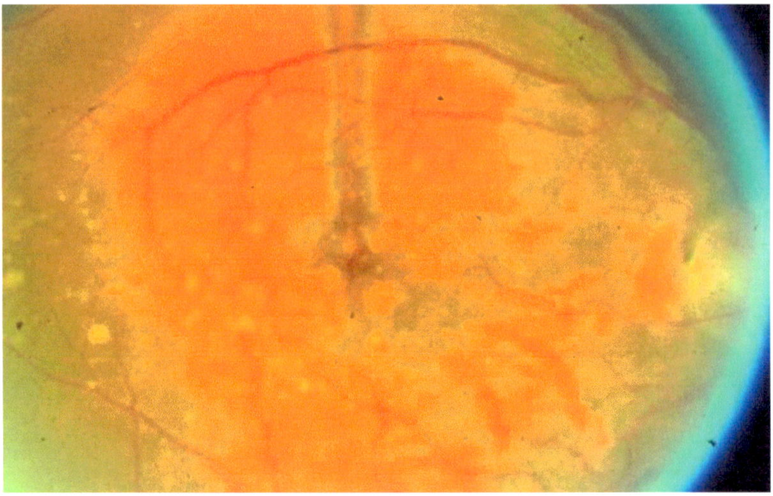

Figure 172 Multiple soft drusen

The prognosis for central vision for this right eye is concerning, although visual acuity was still good. There are numerous drusen, they have various sizes, and the larger ones, fairly close to the foveal center, have very indistinct borders. (The dark vertical lines are artefacts, caused by the pointer in the camera.)

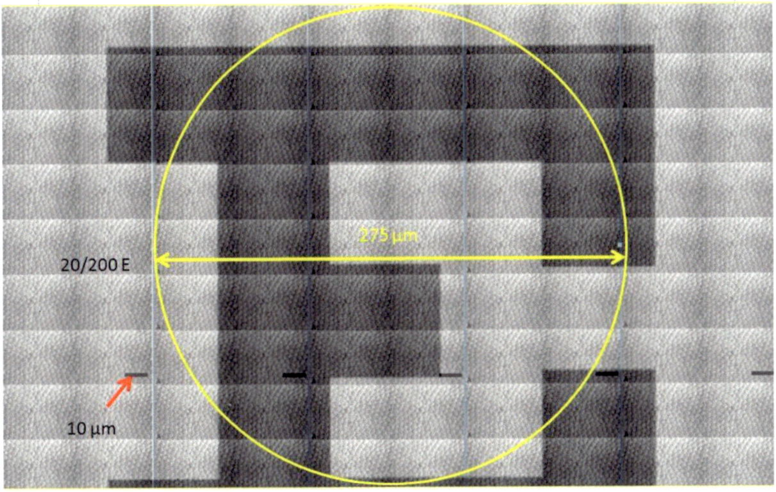


Figure 173 Size of lobule related to 20/200 E

The mosaic of cones is shown here in the background. The black bars represent 10 micrometers, to give a sense of scale. The average size of the lobules of the choriocapillaris (the specific part of the choroid which nourishes the foveal photoreceptors, and is their sole blood supply) is around 275 micrometers, which matches fairly closely the size of the 20/200 E shown in the picture. The 20/200 E is just a little smaller than one degree.

If a typical lobule fails, this is the area of retina which could be affected and make it impossible to recognize the 20/200 E; however, the lobules are of variable size and shape. If this person were to look just to the side of the letters, it would be possible to read them. At worst, macular degeneration affects only ten degrees of central vision, with no effect on the remaining 120 degrees.

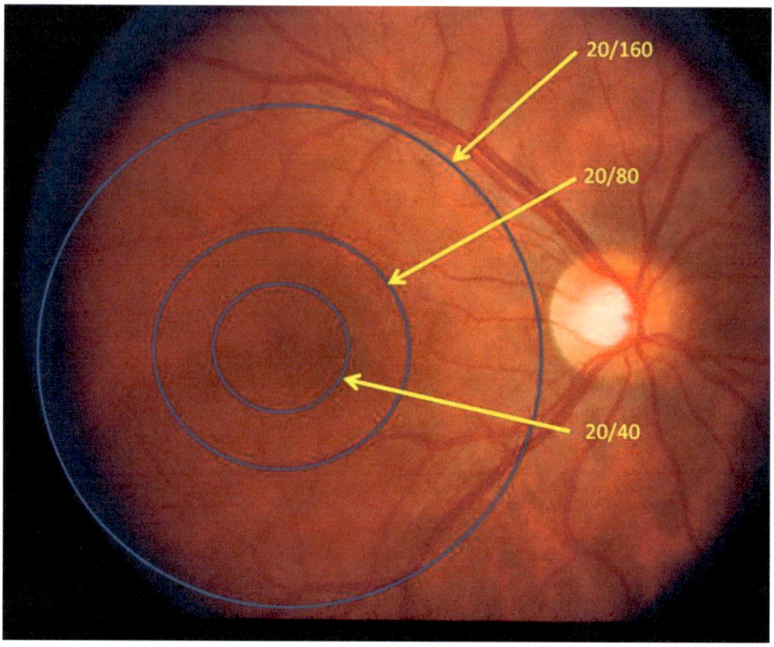


Figure 174 Visual Acuity at various distances from foveal center

The size of a lobule compared to the size of the 20/200 E in Figure 173 is concerning; however, if we consider the visual acuity at various distances from the foveal center, we can see that the loss of the central 1 degree of retina may very well leave a visual acuity better than 20/40. The edge of the lobule shown above in Figure 171 is at a distance of 0.5 degree from the foveal center. Even at a distance of 2.5 degrees (half a nerve head diameter, or 750 micrometers) from foveal center, the visual acuity is still 20/40.

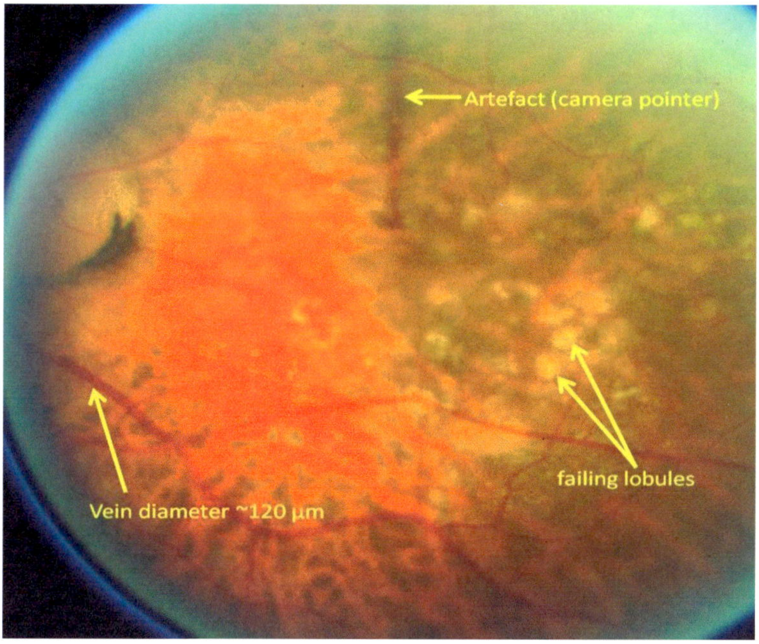


Figure 175 Age related macular degeneration: visual acuity still good

Here is a view of the left eye of a patient with dry age-related macular degeneration. The pigment in the macular area is uneven, with numerous whitish areas, many of which are roughly twice the width of the retinal vein at the left (closer to the nerve head). This agrees with the 275 micrometer estimate of lobule size. When the lobule is failing, the retinal pigment epithelium (RPE) and overlying retina begin to fail as well. Drusen may form, further altering the retinal pigment epithelium. RPE cells with decreased pigment may still be functional. Visual acuity was still 20/40 for this person, and it remained so for nine years. The rest of the retinal appearance is somewhat tiger-striped. Such a striped appearance is normal: this is because the patient had relatively little pigment in the retinal pigment epithelial layer, and lots of pigment in the choroid. The darker choroidal pigment is visible between the salmon-colored choroidal blood vessels.

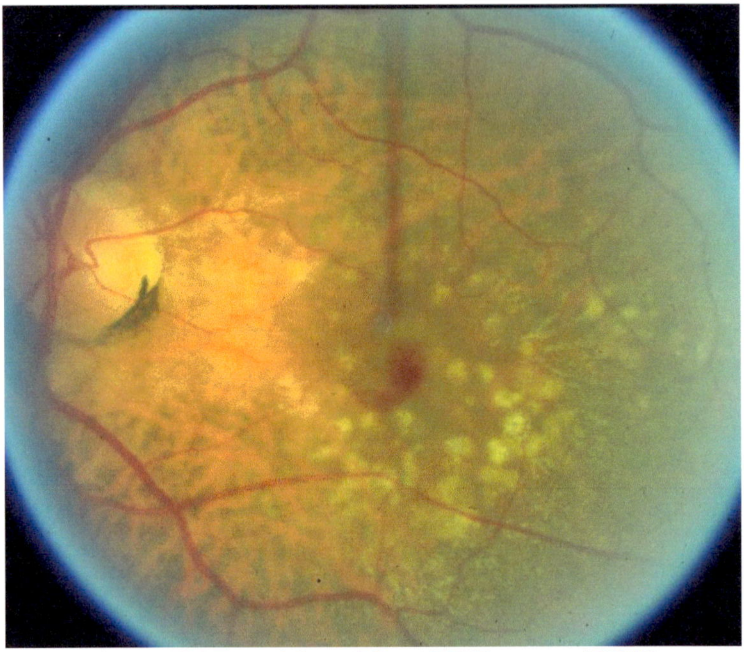

**Figure 176 Transition of dry ARMD to wet ARMD**

Nine years after the photo shown in Figure 175, the patient experienced a decrease in visual acuity and disturbances in her Amsler grid results. The macular degeneration is changing from the dry form to the wet form, as evidenced by the small hemorrhage visible just below the tip of the pointer (dark shadow running into the picture from the top), and the more blurry appearance of the retina around the hemorrhage. In the wet form of macular degeneration, new blood vessels are forming within or below the retina. These new blood vessels have a tendency to leak fluid into the tissues, and can bleed easily. Not all people with dry macular degeneration will progress to the wet form. Regular checking at home with an Amsler grid will give warning of such a change, and then proper treatment must be started promptly. This treatment may consist of intraocular injections of monoclonal antibodies such as Avastin, which interfere with the growth of new blood vessels within the eye.

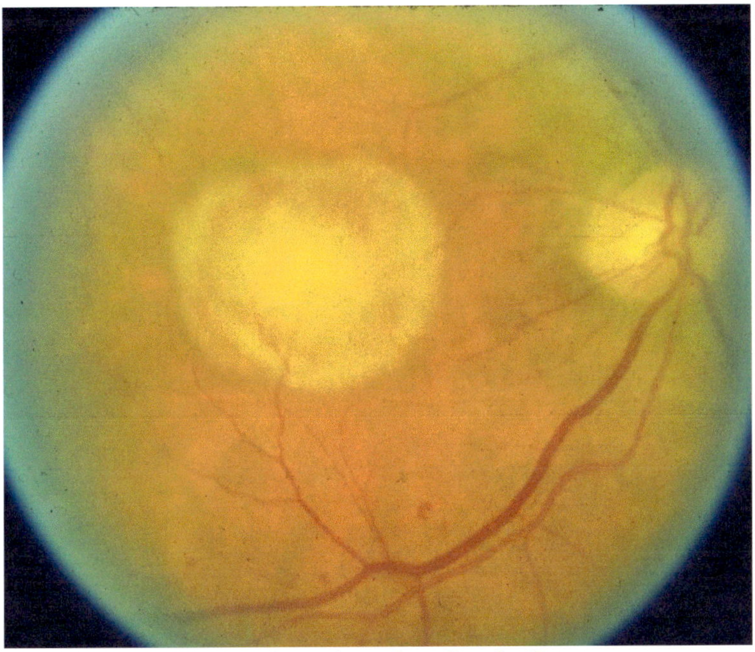

Figure 177 Scar tissue in subretinal space

This patient had a bleed from the choriocapillaris into the space under the retina. What is visible here is scar tissue under the retina. Sadly, the central vision for this person is lost. Considering that the nerve head is about 5 degrees across, we can see that the width of vision loss will be just over 10 degrees wide. In Figure 174, you can see that the visual acuity at the edge of this scarred area (5 degrees from the foveal center) could be 20/80. With the use of magnifying visual aids, this could be substantially improved.

**CONCLUSION**

Now you know more about how the eye works, from its embryonic beginnings to the problems people may have with their eyes throughout their lifetime. Along the way, you have seen how light triggers the visual process and how light can be bent in various ways to help people with their vision. As far as your eye's focus is concerned, there is little difference between light coming from the stars and light coming from only 20 feet away. The dimensions of the eye and its structures range from the thickness of cell membranes (7 nanometers) to the size of the eye itself (which is still only about an inch from front to back). The retina may be only the size of two postage stamps, but its 105 million receptors bring to your brain the whole universe and everything it contains. It takes a galaxy to know another galaxy

# Chapter 9 ABOUT RECEPTORS

Let's think about a cell as though it were a person. If you stepped outside, you might hold up a finger to see how the wind was blowing or a hand to tell if it was raining. If you are thinking about a dip in the ocean, you would probably put a toe in first. The cells of the body are like that: they all have ways of keeping themselves informed about their surroundings.

Some cells in the body are specialized to pick up particular kinds of information; for example, the hair cells in the ear can tell what frequencies of sound are hitting the ear; the photoreceptors of the retina can tell whether there is light hitting the eye; other cells in the middle ear can tell you which way is up.

The finger-like sensors of your cells are called cilia.

Cilia are thought to have evolved some 850 million years ago, before the split between plants and animals.

All cilia are connected to their cell body by a set of nine pairs of microtubules (mobile cilia have ten): the microtubules are involved in transport of proteins, secretions, and other material. Cilia which have a tenth pair of microtubules are able to wave, which is how ependymal cells within the brain help move fluid around, how sperm cells can swim, and how photoreceptor outer segments can move into the best orientation to catch photons.

For the light-sensitive cells of the eye (the photoreceptors), light has to be absorbed by pigment. Basically, no pigment, no light perception. Luckily for us, our eyes have three different kinds of pigment: each one has a 'preference' for its own wavelength. We have some photoreceptors which are particularly sensitive to red, some which respond to blue, and still others which respond to green.

## ACKNOWLEDGEMENTS

I thank Sanjay Agarwal for his professional advice, Gary Fairfoul and Sonny Taylor for their longstanding friendship and encouragement, and Carol Brayman, who suggested I begin a project like this ten years ago, little knowing my penchant for infinite digressions: I am grateful to her for both her patience and editorial skills.

# LIST OF FIGURES

# GLOSSARY

## A

**Accommodation**: a series of events started when you change your interest from a distant object to a near one. The eyes converge, the pupil constricts, and the lens takes a more steeply curved shape to increase its focal power.

**Aneurysm:** in the case of diabetes of long standing (say 10 years or so), these small bulges may occur in the walls of capillaries of the retina. Such aneurysms within the retina are often filled with blood platelets, which closes them off. Aneurysms of major blood vessels can be a major concern, as they may compress adjacent structures: for example, this is the case with aneurysm of the internal carotid artery adjacent to the chiasm.

**Angle kappa (κ):** the angle between the line of sight and the optical axis of the eye. The optical axis is slightly temporal to the line of sight.

**Angle eta (η):** the threshold of stereopsis. The minimum angular difference between two objects which can be detected by using the two eyes together.

**Aqueous humor:** a fluid secreted by the ciliary processes of the ciliary body. Its composition is similar to that of the blood; however, aqueous humor has very little protein (less than 1% of that in blood), and lots of vitamin C (33 times the amount in the blood).

**Artery:** a blood vessel carrying oxygenated blood to the tissues, which may range in size from the aorta (around 30 millimeters) to 0.1 millimeter (100 micrometers). At 150 micrometers, the diameter of the central retinal artery is closer to that of an arteriole.

**Arteriole:** a blood vessel carrying oxygenated blood to the tissues, which may range in size from 0.1 millimeter to 0.035 millimeter (100 to 35 micrometers).

**Aqueous humor:** a fluid secreted by the ciliary processes of the ciliary body. Its composition is similar to that of the blood; however, aqueous humor has very little protein (less than 1% of that in blood), and lots of vitamin C (33 times the amount in the blood).

**Artificial tears:** a tear supplement, consisting of a tear substitute and an agent which can lie on top of the precorneal film to prevent evaporation. If frequent use is necessary, it may be advisable to choose an artificial tear without a preservative.

**Astigmatism:** the focal power of the eye is not the same in (for example) the vertical meridian as it is in (for example) the horizontal meridian. The astigmatic eye cannot produce a point image of a point object, but instead produces two line images for each point on an object.

**Astroglial cell (astrocyte):** In the central nervous system, astroglial cells outnumber neurons. Astrocytes make up half the bulk of the optic nerve head. These glial cells assist in transfer of nutrients from vascular tissue to nerve tissue and constitute the blood/brain barrier.

**Axon:** part of a nerve cell which carries electrical impulses away from the cell body.

**Axoplasm:** a substance produced by the cell body of neurons and transported along the axon toward its termination (orthograde axoplasmic transport) or toward its cell body (retrograde axoplasmic transport). Both forms of transport are necessary for the health of the neuron and for the health of other neurons connected to it.

**B**

**Bipolar cell:** a neuron with a short axon and dendrite. Its dendrite receives information from the photoreceptor, and passes it along its axon to the ganglion cell.

**Blind Spot:** a non-seeing area of the normal visual field found at 15 degrees temporal from the straight-ahead position.

**Bowman membrane:** a layer which lies between the corneal epithelium and the corneal stroma. If it is damaged (for example due to trauma or infection), there will be some residual scar tissue in the cornea.

**Bruch membrane:** an elastic membrane which lies between the retinal pigment epithelium and the choriocapillaris. Portions of Bruch membrane are secreted by the retinal pigment epithelial cells.

## C

**Capillary:** the finest blood vessel in the arteriovenous system. It receives arterial blood from the smallest arteriole. Its wall consists of a single layer of endothelial cells. Its diameter is typically around 6 micrometers, which means that red blood cells, with a diameter of around 7 micrometers, have to squeeze their way through the capillary.

**Capsule:** the elastic envelope surrounding the lens of the eye. Around the equator of the lens, many fibers from the ciliary body attach to the capsule: because of these fibers, the ciliary muscle is able to control the amount of tension on the capsule. More tension causes the lens to be pulled into a flatter shape; less tension allows the capsule to squeeze the lens into a rounder shape.

**Cataract:** this term is best used when opacities in the lens are interfering with life activities. Otherwise, it is better to just talk about lens opacities. These may be present at birth, or develop during life. Opacities may be found in any location in the lens.

**Central Nervous System (CNS):** the brain plus the spinal cord make up the CNS

.

**Cerebrospinal fluid (CSF):** this fluid is found in the ventricles of the brain and surrounds the brain and spinal cord. It is produced by vascular tufts within the ventricles of the brain, in the same manner that aqueous humor is produced in the eye. If there is blockage in the drainage of CSF, raised intracranial pressure results.

**Chiasm:** named after the Greek letter chi (X). This is the area in which half of the Ganglion Cell Axons from each eye cross over to the other side of the brain. Because the crossing axons come from the nasal retina, disturbances of the chiasm tend to cause problems in the temporal visual field. The pituitary gland lies just below the chiasm, while the internal carotid arteries lie close to the lateral sides of the chiasm.

**Choriocapillaris:** the layer of merged capillaries which lies beneath the retina. Outside the choriocapillaris lies the choroid, which supplies it with a generous blood supply.

**Chorioretinitis:** an inflammation of the inner layers of the eye which begins in the choroid. The retina is inflamed, but as a bystander.

**Choroid:** the highly vascular middle layer of the eye.

**Choroiditis:** inflammation of the choroid. See entry for **Cyclitis**.

**Cilia:** (singular cilium) finger-like protrusions from all cells which aid in sensing conditions surrounding the cell. All cilia are anchored to their cell bodies by a set of 9 pairs of microtubules. Some cells (for example, ependymal cells and sperm cells) have 10 pairs and are capable of movement.

**Ciliary Body:** the highly vascular and muscular structure at the front of the eye. The iris is attached to it, the lens is suspended from it, and the ciliary processes (which produce aqueous humor) are attached to it as well.

**Circadian rhythm:** see Diurnal cycle

**Collagen:** a protein found in the cornea and vitreous, as well as elsewhere in the body. With age, the collagen of the vitreous tends to bind together, squeezing out the watery part of the vitreous.

**Conjunctiva:** a thin epithelial layer which lines the back surface of the lid and continues over the surface of the sclera to blend with the epithelium of the cornea at the limbus.

**Cornea:** consists of three layers. The outermost is the epithelium, which is similar to the epithelium all over the body. The middle layer (which makes up most of the corneal thickness) is the **stroma**, which is continuous with the sclera. The innermost layer is the **endothelium**, which is one cell thick, and has the job of pumping water out of the cornea to maintain its transparency.

**Critical angle:** for light travelling from a dense to a rare medium, any rays with an angle of incidence greater than the critical angle will be reflected form the surface. Rays with a lesser angle of incidence will pass through the interface.

**Cyclitis:** inflammation of the ciliary body. Because the ciliary body, iris, and choroid are continuous with each other, it is possible for inflammation of any one of these structures to be accompanied by inflammation of the others. If the ciliary body is inflamed, production of aqueous humor may be reduced, causing reduced intraocular pressure.

## D

**Dendrite:** part of a nerve cell which carries electrical impulses toward the cell body.

**Descemet membrane:** a very tough layer which lies between the endothelial cells at the back surface of the cornea and the corneal stroma. It is a product of the endothelial cells of the cornea.

**Deuteranomalous color vision:** a color vision deficiency caused by a reduced number of green cones.

**Deuteranopia:** the condition of having no green cones.

**Diopter:** the unit of focal power of a lens. For a lens in air, the focal power is the reciprocal of its focal length, measured in meters.

**Diurnal cycle:** many body functions are more or less synchronized with the day/night cycle. These include body temperature, blood pressure, and intraocular pressure, among others.

**Drusen:** bumps on Bruch membrane which cause a thinning of the retinal pigment epithelium, giving the appearance of yellowish spots on the retina.

## E

**Ectoderm:** one of the three layers of the developing embryo. Very early in embryonic development, the ectoderm divides into surface ectoderm and neuroectoderm. For the eye, surface ectoderm gives rise to the top layer of the cornea (epithelium) and the lens. For the eye, neuroectoderm gives rise to the retina and the two back layers of the iris.

**Emmetropia, emmetropic:** if a person can see clearly at distance with no lenses and the eye relaxed, they are emmetropic. The noun for this condition is emmetropia. For the emmetropic eye, parallel rays from a distant object are focused on the retina.

**Endoderm:** the third layer of the developing embryo, which contributes the respiratory and digestive systems.

**Endothelium:** a layer of cells on the back surface of the cornea. These cells are responsible for pumping water out of the cornea so it will remain transparent. Endothelium is also found lining all blood vessels of the body, the subarachnoid space and all lymphatic vessels. The walls of capillaries are made of a single thickness of endothelial cells.

**Entoptic:** a visual experience which arises because of the structure of the eye, rather than from normal stimulation by light.

**Ependymal cell:** a ciliated cell which lines the hollow portions of the entire central nervous system. During embryonic development, ependymal cells are carried into the optic vesicle, where their cilia are modified to become the outer segments of the retinal photoreceptors. After the embryonic stage, the cilia of ependymal cells lining the central nervous system are responsible for moving cerebrospinal fluid around.

**External limiting membrane:** a layer produced by the Mueller cells of the retina. The inner and outer segments of the photoreceptors extend through the external limiting membrane to insert into the retinal pigment epithelium.

F

**Focal length:** distance from a lens to the point at which it will focus rays from a distant object.

**Fovea**: the part of the retina with the sharpest vision. The central portion of the fovea contains only cone photoreceptors.

**Foveal avascular zone (FAZ):** an area about 500 micrometers wide at the foveal center in which the retina has no intraretinal capillaries. The foveal cones are able to provide clearer vision without the interference of the capillaries. The foveal center is entirely dependent on the choriocapillaris for its nourishment.

**Foveola:** a smaller pit at the center of the fovea.

G

**Ganglion cell:** the output neuron for the retina, which gathers data from all other retinal cells (rods, cones, bipolar, horizontal, and amacrine cells) and forwards information to the lateral geniculate body in the midbrain.

**Glaucoma:** a disease in which there is an imbalance between the pressure inside the eye (the intraocular pressure or IOP) and the pressure in the blood vessels nourishing the Optic Nerve Head region. If either the IOP is too high or the blood pressure in the nerve head region is too low, axons of the optic nerve begin to die. Because there are so many axons, and because these pressure changes can develop very gradually, the disease may be present for some years before the loss of axons is detectable. Mechanical effects of raised intraocular pressure may contribute to this disease, by causing stretching of axons and related astroglial cells. Various clinical measurements can assist in detecting glaucoma. These include visual field testing and measurement of thickness of the nerve fiber layer of the retina.

**Glial cell:** a group of supportive cells found in the nervous system. Glial cells are not neurons. In the brain, they outnumber the neurons. This group of cells includes the Mueller cells of the retina, Schwann cells, oligodendrocytes, microglial cells, astrocytes, and ependymal cells.

**H**

**Hemorrhage:** release of blood from a blood vessel. Small hemorrhages in the retina are reabsorbed within two weeks; recurring hemorrhages in the retina are suggestive of an underlying systemic disease, such as anemia.

**Histoplasmosis:** an infection due to *Histoplasma capsulatum,* a fungus common in farming communities and river valley areas. Most infections are minor, but in a few cases, the fungus reaches the retina, where it causes a low-grade inflammatory response.

**Hyalocyte:** a phagocytic cell found in the vitreous humor. It removes foreign matter (such as inflammatory or other cells) which enter the vitreous.

**Hyperopia, Hyperopic:** the eye has a focal power less than it needs, with the result that images tend to fall behind the retina and are seen blurred.

**I**

**Inflammation:** the reaction of the body to injury. The classical signs of inflammation are (1) redness, (2) swelling, (3) pain, (4) decreased function.

**Internal limiting membrane:** a layer produced by the Mueller cells of the retina, which separates the retina from the vitreous.

**Intraocular pressure (IOP):** the eye has a steady production and drainage of aqueous humor. The balance between these two factors determines the pressure within the eye, which is measured in millimeters of mercury (mmHg), the same units used for blood pressure measurement. Normal range of IOP is 10-20 mmHg. If the balance between IOP and the blood pressure in the choroidal vessels supplying the Optic Nerve Head is abnormal (high IOP, low choroidal blood pressure, or both), glaucoma results.

**Iritis:** inflammation of the iris. Iris muscle activity aggravates the pain associated with iritis, leading to avoidance of light (photophobia). See entry for **Cyclitis**.

## J

**Jaundice:** in liver disease, there is an excess of bilirubin (a yellowish pigment) in the blood. While this pigment will appear in the skin in cases of jaundice, the yellow pigment may make an early appearance in the conjunctiva. The strong reflectance of the sclera will make this pigment readily noticeable.

## K

**Keratitis:** inflammation of the cornea.,

## L

**Lamina cribrosa:** a sieve-like area of the sclera at the Optic Nerve Head which allows bundles of Ganglion Cell Axons to pass out of the eye to form the optic nerve.

**Laser:** two types of laser may be used in eye care, depending on the problem. Where there is growth of undesired blood vessels in cases of diabetes, an Argon laser is used: it produces heat to coagulate tissue. Where there is opacification of the lens capsule following cataract surgery, a YAG (Yttrium Aluminum Garnet) laser is used to cause mechanical disruption of the opaque lens capsule.

**Lateral geniculate body (LGB):** located in the middle of the brain, this is a way-station for visual information. At the LGB, axons from the retinal ganglion cells connect with the optic radiation fibers which carry the visual information the rest of the way to the visual cortex at the back of the head.

**Letter acuity:** the ability to read letters on the eye chart of a certain size. If your letter acuity is 20/20, you are able to read from a distance of 20 feet what the average observer can read from a distance of 20 feet. For metric notation, 20/20 is equivalent to 6/6, as 20 feet is roughly equal to 6 meters. If your letter acuity is 20/200, this means that you can read from a distance of 20 feet what the average observer can read from a distance of 200 feet.

**Limbic system:** a part of the brain which lies between the brain stem and the cortex. The limbic system is involved with emotion, learning, motivation, and memory. The hippocampus is part of the limbic system and is an area where new brain cell formation is particularly stimulated by learning.

**Lobule:** the choriocapillaris is composed of subunits called lobules. Each lobule is around 275 micrometers in diameter, and receives arterial blood from the larger arteries of the choroid. This arterial blood travels from the center of the lobule to its periphery, where it drains into the larger veins of the choroid.

## M

**Macular degeneration:** changes in the retina, usually due to decreased blood supply. The retinal pigment epithelium and the overlying photoreceptors are damaged, resulting in decreased visual acuity and loss of portions of the central visual field. In the majority of cases (dry macular degeneration), these losses may take years to develop; in a smaller number, there is growth of new blood vessels which are leaky (wet macular degeneration), and sudden visual changes. Other than measures to improve general health (control of blood pressure and blood sugar levels), there is no specific treatment for dry macular degeneration. Vitamin and dietary supplements may help slow progress of macular degeneration. In the case of wet macular degeneration, specific treatment to deal with new blood vessels formation is useful.

**Melanopsin:** a photopigment found in some retinal ganglion cells. These ganglion cells respond to the overall amount of light striking the retina, and assist in establishing a diurnal (day/night) cycle.

**Meninges:** three layers which surround structures of the central nervous system. The innermost layer is the vascular PIA; the next layer is the ARACHNOID; the outermost layer is the DURA. The meninges cover the brain. They also cover the optic nerve, which shows it is really a TRACT of the central nervous system.

**Mesoderm:** this is the middle layer of the embryo, and gives rise to the circulatory systems, skeleton, and muscles.

**Meter:** the base unit of length in the metric system. 1 meter = 39.37 inches.

**Micrometer (µm) also known as micron:** one thousandth of a millimeter (meter x $10^{-6}$)

**Microscope:** an optical device giving a magnified view of nearby objects. Light rays entering the microscope are diverging, while those emerging from microscope are parallel to each other.

**Millisecond (ms):** one thousandth of a second (second x $10^{-3}$)

**Millimeter (mm):** one thousandth of a meter (meter x $10^{-3}$). One inch = 25.4 millimeters.

**Minimum angle of resolution (MAR):** the theoretical limit of resolution for the human eye, usually considered to be an angle equal to one minute of arc (1/60 of a degree). The most demanding letters for visual acuity charts usually have each of their parts one minute in size. So the famous 20/20 'E' on the eye chart has each of its parts one minute in size, and the size of the whole letter is five minutes.

**Mitochondrion (plural mitochondria):** the main energy source for cells. Mitochondria have a diameter of about 1 micrometer: if they swell (due to decreased oxygen levels, for example), they will begin to scatter light. This is the cause for immediate clouding of the retina in cases of decreased blood supply.

**Mueller cell:** a glial (non-neural) cell of the retina which runs through the thickness of the retina and produces the internal and external limiting membranes. Except for the Optic Nerve Head and foveal region, the Mueller cells provide structural strength. Mueller cells are absent in the nerve head area, making it vulnerable to swelling. Mueller cells lie almost parallel to the retinal surface in the foveal region, and so have difficulty holding the retina together when there is excess fluid in the retina. The Mueller cell also produces strands of collagen which run from the internal limiting membrane into the vitreous.

**Multiple sclerosis:** a condition in which the body's immune system damages myelin, the insulating substance surrounding nerves. Optic neuritis is sometimes an early sign of multiple sclerosis.

**Myopia, Myopic:** the eye has a focal power greater than it needs, with the result that images tend to fall ahead of the retina and be seen blurred. Some eyes may be myopic because of a greater length of the eyeball. In some cases, this may increase the risk of retinal detachment.

**N**

**Nanometer (nm):** one thousandth of a micrometer (meter x $10^{-9}$)

**Neural Crest:** a group of cells derived from the neural tube which are found on the dorsal side of the neural tube after it closes. All pigment cells in the body are derived from the neural crest, with the exception of the retinal pigment epithelium.

**Neuron:** a cell of the nervous system, consisting of a cell body, dendrites, and an axon. Typically, the dendrites carry information to the cell body, and the axon carries information away from the cell body.

**Neuroretina:** the inner layer of the two retinal layers. It contains the photoreceptors and the necessary connections to relay visual information to the brain. Those connections include the bipolar and ganglion cells, and the axons of the ganglion cells which make up the optic nerve.

**Nodal points:** a ray passing through the first Nodal Point (N) emerges from the optical system from the second Nodal Point (N'), with its direction changed.

**O**

**OD and OS:** Oculus Dexter and Oculus Sinister--in other words, right eye and left eye (more eye-related Latin shorthand)

**Oligodendrocyte:** a glial cell found in the central nervous system. Like the Schwann cell of the peripheral nervous system, it provides insulation of axons; however, unlike the Schwann cell, the oligodendrocyte cannot help regeneration of damaged central neurons.

**Optic Cup:** during embryonic development, the optic cup is an outpouching from the developing brain which gives rise to the eye. At the rear of the eye, the inner layer of the optic cup develops into the retina, while the outer layer develops into the retinal pigment epithelium. At the front of the eye, the two layers give rise to the rear two pigmented layers of the iris.

**Optic Nerve Head:** also known as the optic disc, this is the beginning of the optic nerve. Here the million Ganglion Cell Axons leave the eye to form the Optic Nerve Head. Here the central retinal artery enters the eye and the central retinal vein leaves the eye. These vessels supply the retina. By definition, the Optic Nerve Head is the portion of the optic nerve which lies ahead of the lamina cribrosa. Within the Optic Nerve Head, there is usually a depression called the cupping (not to be confused with the optic cup). The nerve head cupping is of variable depth, being nearly flat in some people and quite deep in others. There are no photoreceptors in the optic nerve head, which is why there is a corresponding non-seeing area (the blind spot) in the visual field.

**Optic neuritis:** inflammation of the optic nerve. Because the optic nerve has a rich blood supply, there is a tendency of the tissue to swell; because the optic nerve is contained within the rigid dura of the brain, this swelling tends to cause compression of the optic nerve. This can cause a rapid loss of vision. There are many toxic, infectious, and immunological causes for optic neuritis.

**Optic radiation fiber:** the axon travelling to the visual cortex from its cell body in the lateral geniculate body of the midbrain.

## P

**Papilledema:** swelling of the Optic Nerve Head. This may occur in cases of severe high blood pressure or in cases of increased intracranial pressure.

**Phagocytosis:** a process by which a cell (**phagocyte**) takes material inside its cell membrane and digests it. Histiocytes are phagocytic cells found in all tissues of the body; their opposite number in the central nervous system is the microglial cell. Retinal pigment epithelial cells consume worn-out photoreceptor membranes in the retina, and may wander into the retina proper to work along with microglial cells to remove foreign materials. Phagocytosis is a prime function of white blood cells such as neutrophils and monocytes. Keratocytes, found in the cornea may be transformed into phagocytes. The same is true for hyalocytes, found in the vitreous.

**Photon:** particle of visible electromagnetic radiation produced by the sun or other light sources. A ray of light may be regarded as a stream of photons.

**Photophobia**: the need to avoid bright light. This is particularly marked when there is irritation or inflammation of the iris.

**Photopigment:** a combination of a protein (OPSIN) and a light-sensitive vitamin A compound (RETINAL). When photopigment captures a photon, the RETINAL changes its shape, causing the photoreceptor to send signals to its axon, starting the visual process. The vitamin A compound detaches from the opsin and travels to the retinal pigment epithelial cell where it is converted back to its original shape, which is then recycled to the outer segment to rejoin opsin. Melanopsin is a photopigment found in some retinal ganglion cells. Such ganglion cells are involved in establishing the normal day/night cycles of the body.

**Photopsia:** seeing flashes of light due to mechanical stimulation of the retina. This may routinely occur when the eye is rubbed. Other causes include vitreous detachment, retinal detachment, and macular degeneration.

**Photoreceptor:** a cell of the central nervous system which contains photopigment. When this pigment absorbs light, there are electrical changes in the cell membrane of the photoreceptor.

**Picometer (pm):** one thousandth of a nanometer (meter x $10^{-12}$ )

**Pituitary gland:** a major control center for hormones in the body. It lies just below the chiasm. Tumors of the pituitary gland may cause compression of the lower part of the chiasm.

**Precorneal film:** a layer of mucus, tears, and oil which lies on top of the corneal epithelium. The precorneal film is necessary for the health and optical function of the cornea.

**Presbyopia:** literally means 'old eye'. In clinical terms, this is caused by a sufficient decrease in the plasticity of the crystalline lens that the patient can no longer comfortably read at their preferred reading distance (typically around 40 cm or 16 inches).

**Protanomalous color vision:** a color vision deficiency caused by a reduced number of red cones.

**Protanopia:** the condition of having no red cones

## Q

**Quadrant:** this has two meanings, depending on whether you are talking about the retina or visual field. Quadrants for the retina are divided by two imaginary lines passing horizontally and vertically through the nerve head. For the visual field, quadrants are divided by similar lines, but passing through the fixation point.

## R

**Radiation fiber (also called Optic Radiation fiber:** the axon travelling to the visual cortex from its cell body in the lateral geniculate body in the midbrain. The optic radiation fiber makes a detour into the temporal lobe of the brain on its way around the lateral ventricle of the brain to reach the visual cortex

**Refraction:** bending of light rays when they travel between media of different refractive indices.

**Retinal detachment:** a separation of the receptor outer segments from the retinal pigment epithelium. This will cause some degree of visual impairment, depending on the width of the separation and its location.

**Retinal Pigment Epithelium (RPE):** the outer layer

of the two retinal layers. Its cells are vital to the health of the photoreceptors, and recycle the vitamin A part of photopigment so that the photoreceptors will continue to respond to light. RPE cells have a wide repertoire of actions, including phagocytosis, migration, hyperplasia, and metaplasia.

**Retinochoroiditis:** an inflammation of the inner layers of the eye which begins in the retina. The choroid is involved as a bystander.

**S**

**Schwann cell:** a glial cell found in the peripheral nervous system. It has the responsibility of wrapping itself around the axon of a neuron to produce an insulating layer called myelin. Myelin facilitates the conduction of nervous impulses. The more heavily insulated the axon, the faster it conducts impulses. The Schwann cell is able to help regeneration of damaged peripheral neurons.

**Scotoma:** an area of the visual field where objects are not seen.

**Spectral sensitivity:** in daylight conditions, the retina is most sensitive to yellow-green light (wavelength 555 nanometers). At night, the retina is most sensitive to a wavelength of 507 nanometers (a blue-green color).

**Stereopsis, Stereo acuity:** the ability to see, using our two eyes, that two objects are at different distances from us. Generally, this acuity is better than predicted by letter acuity.

**Stigmatic:** an optical system which is capable of

producing a point image of a point object.

**Subarachnoid space:** the space between the middle covering of the central nervous system (arachnoid) and the innermost covering of the central nervous system (pia). Cerebrospinal fluid flows in the subarachnoid space, and is drained into the venous system.

**Subretinal space:** the space between the receptor outer segments and the retinal pigment epithelium (RPE). Normally, this space is kept very small, due to the RPE constantly pumping fluid out of the space. If there is a break through the thickness of the retina, this will allow fluid from the vitreous side to leak into the subretinal space, resulting in a retinal detachment. If there is too much fluid near the subretinal space, or if the RPE's pumping action is compromised, this may also result in a retinal detachment.

**Synapse:** an area where the axon of one nerve meets with the dendrite of another, with the result that nerve impulses travelling down the axon are transmitted to the dendrite of the next neuron in the chain.

## T

**Telescope:** an optical device giving a magnified view of distant objects. Light rays entering the microscope are parallel to each other, and those emerging are also parallel to each other.

**Threshold:** an imaginary line separating two different places or conditions. The threshold of a room separates it from the adjoining room. When you stand on the threshold, you are (theoretically at least) in neither room. When an object is at the edge of your visual field, it would be visible 50% of the time and invisible the other 50% of the time. See 'Visual Field' under 'FACTS ABOUT YOUR EYE'.

**Toxoplasmosis:** an infection caused by the protozoan *Toxoplasma gondii*, a single-celled organism. Most people have a minor illness, but a few may have damage to the central nervous system, including the retina. This disease can be particularly damaging if the infection reaches a developing fetus.

**Tritanomalous color vision:** a color vision deficiency caused by a reduced number of blue cones.

**Tritanopia:** the condition of having no blue cones.

**U**

**Umbo:** a tiny outward protrusion at the very center of the fovea.

**Uveitis:** a term embracing inflammation of any part of the uveal tract, which includes iris, ciliary body, and choroid. Inflammation of the iris and/or ciliary body is often referred to as anterior uveitis.

## V

**Vernier acuity:** the ability to judge whether or not two lines are lined up with each other. This is the ability which allows us to use vernier calipers. Generally, this acuity is better than predicted by letter acuity.

**Visual Acuity:** usually given as 20/x, where x is the distance at which an average person can see an object, compared to what you can see at 20 feet. For example, if the average observer can see an object at 20 feet and you can too, your visual acuity is 20/20. On the other hand, if the average observer can see an object at 400 feet, and you can only see it from a distance of 20 feet, then your visual acuity is 20/400.

**Visual Cortex:** located at the back of the brain, this is the gray layer of cells which receive input from the eye. The brain consists of white matter (dendrites and axons) and gray matter (cells). The axons of the radiation fibers connect with cells in the visual cortex.

**Visual Field:** the area over which a specified object may be seen by one eye without turning the eye. The size of the visual field depends on variables such as the size of the object, lighting, and how it is moving. Larger, brighter objects are seen further to the side than smaller, dimmer objects. Problems at any point in the visual pathway may have an impact on the visual field.

**Vitreous detachment:** a separation of the outer envelope of the vitreous from the inner limiting membrane of the retina. In many cases, this is a benign, age-related event. If there is a strong attachment between the vitreous and retina, however, a retinal hole could result, with the risk of retinal detachment.

**W**

**Wavelength:** a method of describing electromagnetic radiation. The visible spectrum of light includes wavelengths between 400 (blue) and 700 (red) nanometers (nm). One nanometer is $1 \times 10^{-9}$ meter. In daylight, the human eye is optimally sensitive to the wavelength of 555 nm, a yellowy green. At night, this shifts to 507 nanometers (a blue-green color). The visible spectrum occupies only a tiny range of wavelengths: the whole electromagnetic spectrum ranges from gamma rays (wavelength $< 1 \times 10^{-11}$ meters) to radio waves (some > hundreds of kilometers). Generally, the shorter wavelengths have more energy: in terms of the visible spectrum, the ultraviolet portion has more energy: this is why you can get a sunburn if you are not protected from ultraviolet.

**X**

**Xerosis**: dryness of the skin or body membranes. This may affect the conjunctiva and cornea particularly when there is a shortage of tears. Dry eye may arise because of vitamin A deficiency, or simply because of decreased blinking when you spend a lot of time looking at a computer or other screen. In severe cases of xerosis, bacteria may invade the cornea, causing potential sight loss.

**Y**

**YAG laser:** a YAG (Yttrium Aluminum Garnet) laser is used to cause mechanical disruption of the lens capsule if it becomes opaque following cataract surgery.

**Z**

**Zonule:** collectively, all the fine strands (zonular fibers) running from the ciliary body to the lens capsule are referred to as the zonule.

Made in the USA
Las Vegas, NV
03 November 2026

57423448R00145